THE MALE NURSE

R. G. S. BROWN
and
R. W. H. STONES

OCCASIONAL PAPERS ON SOCIAL ADMINISTRATION. 52
Editorial Committee under the
Chairmanship of Professor B. Abel-Smith
Published by G. Bell & Sons,
York House, Portugal Street, London, W.C.2

First published 1973
© *Copyright 1973 by The Social Administration Research Trust*

ISBN 07135 1879 0 (Case)
ISBN 07135 1878 2 (Limp)

MADE AND PRINTED IN ENGLAND BY
WILLMER BROTHERS LIMITED
BIRKENHEAD

TABLE OF CONTENTS

PAGE

FOREWORD

This series of *Occasional Papers* was started in 1960 to supply the need for a medium of publication for studies in the field of social policy and administration which fell between the two extremes of the short article and the full-length book. Since the inception of this Series of papers, it has, however, been extended to include many which might better be described as books : comparative speed of publication being one factor that has attracted authors to us. It was thought that such a series would not only meet a need among research workers and writers concerned with contemporary social issues, but would also strengthen links between students of the subject and administrators, social workers, committee members and others with responsibilities and interest in the social services.

Many of the papers have been written by members of the Department of Social Science and Administration at the London School of Economics and Political Science. Contributions are, however, welcome from any source and should be submitted in the first instance to the Chairman, The Social Administration Research Trust, at the London School of Economics. A list of some of the earlier papers which are still available is printed on the back of this volume. Copies may be obtained through any bookseller.

Brian Abel-Smith

THE AUTHORS

R. G. S. Brown is Senior Lecturer and R. W. H. Stones was formerly Research Assistant in the Department of Social Administration at the University of Hull.

PREFACE AND ACKNOWLEDGEMENTS

As a result of discussions with the Department of Health and Social Security (then the Ministry of Health) in 1966, it was agreed that it would be useful for the Department of Social Administration at Hull University to study the recruitment and wastage of male entrants to nurse training. The original plan was to interview a number of men soon after they started training in order to obtain information about their background, motivations and expectations, and again a year later to discover their reactions to training and their feelings about a nursing career at that time. It was later decided to supplement the questionnaires with intelligence and personality tests and with information supplied by the training schools. Later still, it was decided to expand the study and follow the entrants' progress up to the completion of their training and for two years beyond.

The first round of interviews took place during 1968 and the second series was arranged in 1969. The sample included about one sixth of all the men who commenced a course of nurse training in England and Wales in 1968. Both general and mental nursing were represented on a range of training programmes whose length varied, according to the circumstances of the trainee and the qualification for which he was aiming, from twelve months to three years with the possibility of extensions to allow for several attempts at the final examination. The first members of the cohort to finish their training did so in June 1969 and the last result was obtained in October 1972. By the end of 1972, therefore, we knew which of the original entrants had successfully completed their training. We also had information about the subsequent careers of nearly all those who had taken the shorter courses. We felt that this gave us a sufficiently clear picture to justify preparing a main report on the survey. The research will not be complete until

1974, when the last qualifier has been followed for two years into his career as a trained nurse. The early material would by then have looked somewhat dated and we considered that it was better to publish the bulk of our results now. The outstanding findings will be published, mainly in the nursing press, as soon as possible after they become available.

This report is concerned with the contribution that men can make to nursing and with difficulties that may prevent it from being fully exploited. After an introductory survey, successive chapters are concerned with the social, educational and personal characteristics of the men in our survey, with the routes through which they came into nurse training, with their self-image, with the difficulties they experienced during their training and with factors affecting their ultimate success and failure. The conclusions in the final chapter support and confirm the recommendations of the Briggs Committee on Nursing, whose report (Cmnd. 5115) was published in October 1972, so far as they concern male nurses. Our main conclusion is that men have a considerable contribution to make to the nursing profession although there are some practical problems to be overcome if full use is to be made of this potential source of recruitment. There is nothing inconsistent or effeminate about the notion of a male nurse. Nursing can offer a satisfying career to men who are dissatisfied with more conventional occupations. But there is a credibility gap to be overcome if potential male recruits and the public at large are to be helped to see nursing as a job for men.

Because of their immediate interest to those concerned with the recruitment and training of nurses in the national health service, some of our findings on specific issues have already been published in short papers which are either preliminary or complementary to the material brought together in this report. The interested reader will find them listed at the end of the volume. We are grateful to the editors of the *Nursing Times,* the *International Journal of Nursing Studies* and *Social and Economic Administration* for permission to reproduce some key passages.

We should like to express our gratitude to the 542 men who allowed themselves to be interviewed and to the senior administrative nursing staff and tutors at 57 different hospitals who not only allowed us to interview these student and pupil nurses but supplied copious material about their training arrangements and about the progress of individual trainees over a long period of time. Without their generous help the survey could not have been carried out. We are also grateful to Mrs Laurie S. Millward, who worked on the research from 1967–70 and was responsible for designing the questionnaires, organizing the interviews and coding the replies; to our interviewers; to Mr M. J. Norman for his assistance with computation; and to Miss Lynda Wright who as secretary to the project maintained the flow of information from hospitals as well as transmuting our rough drafts into readable form. At the design stage we had help and advice from many people including Dr Jillian MacGuire, Dr Sybil Eysenck, Mrs Hilary Leigh, Dr A. G. Davies and Dr Arthur Willcocks. The staff of the General Nursing Council Research Unit were unfailingly helpful and courteous throughout the survey, in particular by obtaining from the Council's inspectorate a confidential and informal assessment of the nurse training school at each hospital in the survey. Our greatest single debt is to Miss H. M. Simpson and her colleagues at the Department of Health and Social Security who provided financial support for the survey and its various extensions, commented helpfully on many draft reports and supplied general support and encouragement.

University of Hull, February 1973

1. INTRODUCTION

In Britain, as in most other industrial societies, nursing is predominantly a female occupation. In 1972 270,293 (89%) of the 304,834 nursing staff in National Health Service hospitals in England and Wales (including auxiliary nurses and nurses in training) were women.[1] The same general pattern is found in other countries; hardly anywhere do women constitute less than three quarters of the nursing labour force.[2] In most countries nursing is one of the major female professions, rivalled only by teaching in the number of women it employs.

Male nurses, therefore, are very much in the minority. This is even more true if we look at fully qualified nurses. Although men are often employed in large numbers as auxiliaries, particularly in mental hospitals, they rarely account for more than ten per cent of professionally trained nurses in any country. England and Wales are fairly exceptional, in that sixteen per cent of qualified nurses are men. In the United States, less than one per cent of professional nurses are male. Some countries, such as Italy, do not even provide full professional nurse training for men.

Nursing is usually described and presented to the public as a job for women. 'The most favoured group [for recruitment] has been very clearly defined. It consists of young unmarried women with middle-class backgrounds, grammar school education and English parentage'.[3] Although in Britain some recruitment material is now aimed specifically at men, nursing is not an obvious first choice of occupation for males. A 1966 survey of English school leavers did not find a single boy who said he intended to take up a career in nursing.[4] Similar findings have been reported from the United States where high school senior boys rated nursing the lowest in terms of masculinity in relation

13

to other comparable occupations.[5] In other cultures, however, especially in the Middle East and South East Asia, nursing is not necessarily a job for women and may even be barred to them.

In its report on the employment and conditions of work of nurses in 1960, the International Labour Office spelled out the basic tasks of nurses as direct care of patients, teaching and administration.[2] There was nothing in this description to suggest that nursing must be a female occupation. The British Royal College of Nursing has pointed out that 'The spectrum of activities encompassed by the generic term "nursing" is so wide that it provides opportunities for those with a variety of aptitudes, abilities and inclinations'.[6] In the words of the 1972 Briggs Committee: 'Not one type of nurse is required, but many'. Although there is still a need for the tender loving care traditionally rendered at the bedside by young female nurses, there are many other demands on nursing staff. The technical advances required to keep pace with medical developments and increasing specialization demand types of ability and aptitude which may be found as readily in men as in women. There is some evidence that male and female nurses have different attitudes to their roles which affect the kind of service they offer. Morris[7] found that male nurses in mental subnormality hospitals tended to emphasize the rehabilitative, custodial and training aspects of their work whereas female nurses laid greater emphasis on basic nursing and patient care. Some have argued that men bring a kind of emotional objectivity and technical ability which is ideally suited to the modern needs of nursing.[8]

Whilst there are sociological reasons (notably its association with maternal care) for the emphasis on nursing as a feminine skill, it is also apparent that the predominantly female composition of the profession in this and other western countries has developed as a result of specific historical circumstances.

EARLY HISTORY OF NURSING

In most ancient civilizations, both Asian and European, the sick were attended almost exclusively by men. It has been recorded that men were assisting doctors in Asia fourteen centuries before Christ; and male servants were employed to look after the sick in ancient Greece. At the time of Hippocrates in the fifth century BC only male assistance is recorded for doctors. Later the crusades saw the emergence of the military nursing orders, the most famous of these being the Knights Hospitallers of St John of Jerusalem.[9] The western tradition of male nursing, in both military and religious orders, lasted several centuries and survives today in the modern lay nursing organizations, notably the St John's Ambulance Brigade and the British Red Cross Society. The code of discipline which characterized the early orders of male nurses was later adopted by the secular nursing orders of

14

women, among them the Béguines in Belgium, which became an outlet for women's activity. The disciplined female nursing force eventually inspired the modern development of nursing in the 19th century.

In England, the foundations of the modern nursing profession were laid by Elizabeth Fry's Sisters of Charity and the Florence Nightingale Training School. But for the first half of the nineteenth century, according to Abel-Smith, 'nursing amounted to little more than a specialized form of charring'.[10]It was performed for the well-to-do by domestic servants and for the poor by fellow-paupers in the workhouses. Nurses in the voluntary hospitals tended to be drawn from among those in domestic service and were nearly all women. There were some men among the 'pauper' nurses and others worked in asylums and as domiciliary mental nurses, many on jobs no female could or would undertake. The reforms initiated by Florence Nightingale in the second half of the century turned what many regarded as a disreputable job into an honourable and respectable profession for women.

One of the most important aspects of this development was that it occurred during a time of female surplus over males, accentuated by losses of men in the Crimea which were to be repeated in the first world war. Employment opportunities for the large numbers of unmarried women were limited and, encouraged by the prospects of independent status, many turned to nursing. For the minority of upper-class 'lady nurses' who became the driving force behind the movement for registration and full professional status, nursing offered power and a relatively rewarding career. It also appealed to the romantic or dedicated type of girl. Moreover the ideals of nursing were in line with the tenets of the High Church movement. Although nursing involved a subordinate role it nevertheless represented a step towards female emancipation.

The leaders of the move for professionalization took full advantage of this. Once it became established that the newly created 'matrons' had undisputed authority over their nursing staff the chance of accepting males as full members of the profession became more remote. Men, it was thought, would be harder to control. There was even some prejudice from doctors who believed that men were more likely than women to usurp their own functions in the voluntary hospitals. Such men as there were in nursing had inferior social origins and were not thought to share the high ideals of the 'lady nurses'.

MALE EMANCIPATION: 1900–1950
Nevertheless in 1901 there were about 5,700 male nurses, performing many of the jobs which women refused. They were not accepted in the voluntary hospitals but were confined to mental institutions and domiciliary work. The only qualification open to them was the certificate

15

which the Royal Medico-Psychological Society instituted for mental nurses in 1891.[11] Mental hospitals were often in the hands of married couples who supervized their respective 'sides'. But from about 1900 onwards overall control began to be assumed by matrons who came from the voluntary general hospitals. They introduced into mental nursing the new regime of rigid discipline and para-military organization, with no lay interference. Chief male nurses lost much of their authority and did not regain equal status until after the inception of the National Health Service.

The position of male nurses was not improved with the introduction of State Registration. When the General Nursing Council and the Register of Nurses were established in 1919 male nurses were put on a separate register which was maintained for thirty years. Male nurses in general hospitals were usually employed only to give VD treatment and although some local authority hospitals began to train men for general nursing, only a hundred or so were being trained in non-mental hospitals by the early 1930s. The apparent prejudice which existed against the male nurse was attributed by Abel Smith to a mixture of 'snobbery and feminism' with a hint of sexual taboos.[12]

Between the wars, a growing shortage of suitable female recruits for general nursing threatened the maintenance of high professional standards. 'Assistant nurses', unqualified and untrained, were employed in general hospitals. But there was still no recourse to male recruitment. Even the 1932 Lancet Commission on Nursing,[13] which considered proposals for remedying the nursing shortage, failed to appreciate the possibilities for men. In the meantime the total number of male nurses was rising and had reached 15,000 by 1931. Recruitment was boosted by the unemployment of the depression years.

During the second world war many men got their first taste of general nursing in the Royal Army Medical Corps. Some of them were recruited into hospitals under special arrangements as Enrolled Assistant Nurses or (after a shortened form of training) as Registered Nurses when the war ended. In some ways the war weakened the prejudice against men: many female nurses had worked alongside male orderlies and realized their potential value in general nursing. By 1950, five years after the end of the war, there were 1,719 male registered nurses in general hospitals, nearly six times the pre-war figure, plus a further 3,000 enrolled assistant nurses. But the war had also 'codified civilian discrimination'[14] against men because female nurses, including many untrained auxiliaries, were automatically given officer status in the Queen Alexandra's Imperial Military Nursing Service while the men in the RAMC generally remained in the ranks.

After the war the Ministry of Health working party on the recruitment and training of nurses[15] reviewed the whole structure of the nursing profession and suggested, in a couple of paragraphs, that all

16

nursing posts be thrown open equally to males and females. The working party recognized however that the success of any scheme for mixing male and female nurses in general hospitals would depend on the reactions both of the profession and of the public.

Official changes followed quickly. Nearly all formal discrimination against men disappeared with the Nurses Act of 1949, which provided for the amalgamation of the male part of the register with the general part. By 1950 there were 25,600 male nurses, trained and untrained, constituting 17 per cent of the total nursing labour force. A quarter of all full-time trained nurses (including enrolled assistant nurses) were men and in mental hospitals there were twice as many trained male as female nurses. But even in mental nursing men accounted for only half the total nursing labour force, owing to the large number of part-time female assistant nurses and the high proportion of female students.

DEVELOPMENTS SINCE 1950

The two decades since 1950 have seen important developments in nursing manpower which have affected the position of male nurses. The demand for nursing staff has greatly increased as a result of the general expansion of services, medical advances, the more intensive use of available beds and the greater dependency of hospital patients on nursing care.

This demand has been met by an increase in the total number of nurses (excluding midwives) in NHS hospitals in England and Wales from almost 152,000 in 1950 to just over 288,000 in 1971. But the composition of distribution of the nursing labour force has been changing in six main ways.[16]

(a) There are more unqualified nursing auxiliaries and assistants: 27% of the 1971 total were unqualified compared with 20% in 1950.

(b) There has been a shift towards part-time working, particularly among female staff: the proportion of female nurses who work part-time increased from 16% in 1950 to 36% (including 41% of registered female nurses) in 1971. This has enabled many married women to return to nursing (over half of married nurses and midwives do so) and replaces some of the loss which occurs when newly-qualified female nurses give up nursing on marriage.

(c) There has also been a very substantial increase in the number of qualified nurses – from 57,000 full-time registered and enrolled nurses and 13,000 part-time in 1950 to 86,000 full-time and 53,000 part-time in 1971.

(d) The number of nurses in training has not risen proportionately: after a peak in the early 1960s the number of students fell back to 1950 levels of approximately 50,000 in 1970 and 1971, although they were augmented by 21,000 pupil nurses. Consequently the ratio of

17

qualified nurses to trainees improved during the period. Nevertheless, even in 1971 a quarter of all hospital nursing staff were trainees (compared with a third in 1950).

(e) There are more enrolled nurses and pupils. Enrolled nurse status is attained after two years practical training as a pupil nurse, compared with the three years student nurse training required for registration. The popularity of the roll increased markedly after the introduction of a minimum educational requirement for student nurse training, first in general and later in psychiatric* hospitals. By 1971, enrolled nurses (including some who had been enrolled under transitional arrangements on the basis of experience) accounted for one qualified nurse in three while pupil nurses comprised nearly a third of nurses in training.

(f) There has been a shift of nursing manpower from psychiatric to general hospitals. In particular, mental illness hospitals have not fully shared in the increase of registered nurses; between 1950 and 1971 their number had increased by only 5% compared to a 62% increase in mental subnormality hospitals and a 79% increase in non-psychiatric hospitals.

Most of these changes are connected with the heavy dependence of nurse staffing on women, many of them recruited from a fairly narrow age-band in their late teens and therefore directly affected by such demographic trends as fluctuations in the birth rate twenty years earlier and the modern habit of early marriage and childbearing, often followed by a return to part-time employment.

The contribution that men have been making to the total nursing situation can best be examined against this background. In fact, although the numbers of qualified and trainee male nurses have been rising steadily, with a sharp increase in the number of trainees in the early 1970s, the total male contribution has declined from 17% of all nursing staff in 1950 to 11% in 1971. But the nature of their contribution is different and in some ways runs contrary to the trends in female nurse staffing. Relatively few men are part-time, which means that they contribute a higher proportion of actual nursing hours than the raw figures suggest. A higher proportion of them are qualified: whereas the ratio of qualified female staff to trainees is about two to one, among male nurses it is nearer three to one. They tend to train for the register rather than for the roll and, possibly because they are drawn from a wider band of age and ability, the number of male students has not been falling off in the same way as females.

It is instructive to look at the last point in more detail, because nurses in training are the qualified nurses of the future. Table 1.1 shows the number of new entrants to nurse training for each year from 1965 to 1971. The annual decline until 1970 in the number of new female

* We have used the term 'psychiatric' hospitals to cover both hospitals for the mentally ill and those for the mentally subnormal. The term 'mental subnormality' (MSN) is used throughout as this was in force at the time of the survey. The official term is now 'mental handicap'.

students is partly counterbalanced by a steady increase in the number of male entrants. Even the sharp increase after 1970 (which probably reflects a temporary shortage of alternative employment for young people) was 62% for males against 21% for females. Consequently the

TABLE 1.1

Numbers of student and pupil nurses starting training in England and Wales for the first time in 1965–71

	1965	1966	1967	1968	1969	1970*	1971*
Student nurses:							
Male	1,512	1,929	2,003	1,885	1,857	2,000	3,232
Female	18,448	17,570	16,981	15,062	14,585	14,277	17,260
Pupil nurses:	7,891	9,920	11,329	11,559	12,105	13,329	16,008
Total	27,851	29,419	30,413	28,506	28,547	29,606	36,600

* year commencing 1st April

Source: GNC statistics — Admissions to the Index of Student Nurses and the Index of Pupil Nurses (annual).

proportion of men among student nurses (at all stages in training) rose from 10.4% in 1965 to 14% in 1970 and 15.5% in 1971, and can be expected to rise even further in the future. (Female entrants, however, accounted for over 90% of the pupil nurses shown in the table.)

The drift away from psychiatric nursing is, if anything, more pronounced for men than for women. The number of registered male nurses in mental illness hospitals has actually been declining during the twenty year period, although the decline has been offset by increases in female registered nurses and enrolled nurses of both sexes. During this period the number of registered male nurses in non-psychiatric hospitals nearly trebled, from 1,700 in 1950 to nearly 5,000

TABLE 1.2

Qualified nurses and nurses in training, by sex and status, in hospitals in England and Wales, 1950–71

			1950	1960	1965	1970	1971
Registered nurses	Males	Full-time	11,124	12,074	12,984	13,906	14,297
		Part-time	48	422	900	1,388	1,410
	Females	Full-time	33,542	42,318	44,082	45,925	46,048
		Part-time	7,478	13,927	20,832	30,094	31,876
Enrolled nurses	Males	Full-time	3,013	1,781	2,829	4,053	4,177
		Part-time	47	74	136	347	340
	Females	Full-time	9,166	8,365	12,637	20,021	20,982
		Part-time	5,251	6,100	9,911	18,367	19,697
Student nurses	Males	Full-time	5,679	5,040	5,264	5,966	6,616
	Females	Full-time	43,738	49,035	50,642	42,680	42,826
Pupil nurses	Males	Full-time	257	234	338	1,566	1,858
		Part-time	—	—	—	2	1
	Females	Full-time	1,991	5,543	10,757	17,960	19,034
		Part-time	—	58	273	939	1,221

Source: DHSS (and Ministry of Health) Hospital Nursing Staff tables.

in 1971. The growth of male students, too, has been much slower in mental illness than in non-psychiatric hospitals, which by 1971 accounted for 37% of all male students. These include post-registration students who are already qualified in psychiatric nursing and are seeking a second qualification – and in some cases a wider career – in general nursing.

The changing numbers of qualified and trainee nurses, by sex and category, are summarized in Table 1.2.

THE STATUS OF MALE NURSES TODAY

The years since the war have seen substantial changes in the position of men in nursing. One effect of the gradual breaking down of sex barriers in western societies is that in this country the only field of nursing barred to men is midwifery. Even here the barriers are coming down and already in Scotland male nurses can take obstetrics as part of their general training. Men can nurse sick children and work on female wards in general hospitals, at the discretion of the hospital authorities. The main London teaching hospitals finally began to admit men for training in 1966. Male nurses are also playing a role in the community. The first male Queen's Nurse began work on the district as far back as 1947 and in 1961 the first men were trained as Health Visiting Officers. (The law is in the process of being changed to allow men to qualify as Health Visitors.) By 1970 about 500 men were employed in local authority nursing services.[17]

Institutionalized prejudice against men within the nursing profession has now almost disappeared. The General Nursing Council included five males out of thirty-one nurses on the full council in March 1972 and a relatively larger male representation on its mental nurses' committee. The Royal College of Nursing (RCN) did not admit male nurses as full members until 1960 but now has a male membership of several thousand, some of whom sit on its Council. In addition, as a result of the many years in which they were barred from full membership of the nurses' main professional body, male nurses have long had their own organizations. Male nurses were originally affiliated to the RCN through the Society of Registered Male Nurses Ltd, founded in 1937, which itself went into liquidation in 1968 having achieved what it set out to do – gain equality in a female environment.[18] Men in psychiatric hospitals still play a large part in the Confederation of Health Service Employees which is represented on the Whitley Council that negotiates salaries for nurses and midwives.

Probably the best indication that men are gaining equality with women is the fact that more opportunities have opened up for male nurses. In psychiatric hospitals the segregation of the sexes has been breaking down and men have taken many of the top posts at the head of integrated nursing services. The introduction of a new standardized grading system for nursing posts, following the recommendations of the Salmon Report on Senior Nursing Staff Structure in 1966,[19] has also opened up opportunities in general hospitals. Not least it has hastened the disappearance of the curious title 'male matron'. By 1972 there were 72 male members of the Association of Nurse Administrators (formerly the Association of Hospital Matrons). In all types of hospitals the number of men in the top two grades of Principal Nursing Officer and Chief Nursing Officer increased eight fold between 1969 and 1972 compared to only a five fold increase for females. In 1972 men occupied a third of all these posts. There was only one female Chief Nursing Officer in a mental hospital.

But the recent opening up of opportunities at the top of the profession does not hide the fact that nursing has offered a relatively unattractive career to men and it is important to look at their position in some detail.

NURSING AS A CAREER FOR MEN

The main disincentives to men would seem to be career and promotion prospects, plus the traditional deterrents associated with nursing – pay and conditions of work, particularly hours. The International Labour Office, reporting in 1960 on the employment and conditions of work of nurses throughout the world, found that nurses generally experienced poor conditions in relation to other occupations,[20] The disadvantages are probably greater for men, who in Britain are paid the same rates as female nurses. The Whitley Council staff

TABLE 1.3

Grades of full-time registered nurses, by sex and field, at
September 1971
(Hospitals, England and Wales)

	All non-psychiatric hospitals	Mental illness	MSN	All hospitals
WOMEN				
No. of whole-time registered nurses	39,402	4,851	1,795	46,048
OF WHOM:				
Staff Nurse	33%	24%	19%	32%
Ward sister*	48%	63%	62%	50%
Higher grades	19%	13%	19%	18%
MEN				
No. of whole-time registered nurses	4,728	6,841	2,728	14,297
OF WHOM:				
Staff Nurse	18%	31%	22%	24%
Charge nurse*	52%	53%	60%	54%
Higher grades	30%	16%	18%	22%

* Including deputy ward sister/charge nurse.

Source: DHSS statistics. Part-time staff are excluded in order to give a better comparison between the career prospects of male and female staff.

side used the low pay of male nurses as a bargaining point in the 1968 pay campaign and invited the Prices and Incomes Board to devise a salary structure which would attract more men. The Board's only positive response to this, however, was to suggest that men training in psychiatric hospitals should be able to claim dependents' allowances.[21] (They also proposed an increase from £50 to £100 for the special salary addition for staff in psychiatric hospitals, and its extension to wider groups of staff of both sexes.)

One reason for the decline in the popularity of psychiatric nursing among men could be that the promotion prospects for male nurses in this field are poorer than those of female nursing staff. For a detailed picture we have to look at the ratio of senior to junior posts for male and female nurses in different types of hospital (see Table 1.3). The table shows that in September 1971 relatively more men than women were holding posts above the basic staff nurse level – and even more markedly above the charge nurse/ward sister level – in the general hospitals. On the other hand proportionately more men than women were in the basic grade in psychiatric hospitals (where most of the men are to be found). There is a marked contrast with the position in 1960 when only 15% of full-time male registered nurses in non-psychiatric hospitals held posts above charge nurse, compared with 30% in 1971 (the percentages for women being 22% and 19%). Over the same period the proportion of men in the higher grades of psychiatric nursing has risen from 12% to 16% while the proportion of women has dropped from 17% to 13%. Superficially, men are doing quite well.

The prospects look less inviting however when age structure, and the fact that most of the men have family responsibilities, are taken into account. After reviewing the age and time in post of men and women in different grades in November 1967, the Prices and Incomes Board commented that the male nursing staff in psychiatric hospitals were older and gave longer service in equivalent grades in general hospitals and that their promotion prospects were much poorer than those of female nursing staff.[22] Taking all hospitals together only 22% of male charge nurses were then under 35 and 51% were 45 or over, whereas 41% of female ward sisters were under 35 and only 35% over 45. Of the male staff nurses, 12% were under 25 and 47% were over 35, whereas 49% of the female staff nurses were under 25 and only 19% over 35. The age differential between men and women held for all trained staff including the enrolled nurse grade. It was partly due to the relative youth of many female nurses in the general hospitals and also to the speed with which the women who stay in nursing move upwards once they are registered. The very absence of wastage among men leads to promotion blockages and causes them to spend longer than women in the staff nurse grade. Summary figures for different types of hospitals are shown in Table 1.4.

22

TABLE 1.4
Age and time in post of registered nurses, by sex and field, in
November 1967 (Great Britain)

Type of Hospital:	Acute general		Mental illness		MSN	
	Male	Female	Male	Female	Male	Female
CHARGE NURSE/WARD SISTER						
– average age (yrs)	41.0	37.0	45.3	44.1	44.3	44.2
– average years in post	6.4	6.0	6.0	7.0	5.5	3.6
STAFF NURSE						
– average age (yrs)	32.5	26.8	36.9	35.8	36.0	34.8
– average years in post	2.2	1.6	6.7	3.0	3.6	2.1

Source: Cmnd. 3585.

Against this, the Salmon investigations suggested that in England and Wales men took less time to reach the higher grades once they had broken through the charge nurse bottleneck.[23] The annual turnover of posts at that level was 12% for women but only 10% for men. Consequently many men were not appointed to the grade until over 40 and once appointed they were more likely to remain in it for over five years. On the other hand fewer men than women spent more than ten years at charge nurse level or in the intermediate grades below Chief Male Nurse/Matron. Half the men who made the top posts did so within ten years of becoming charge nurses, whereas only a third of the women who became Matrons did so within ten years of becoming sisters and 46% took over fifteen years. Men therefore reached the top posts at an earlier age: of those appointed Chief Male Nurse or Matron in 1960–64, 20% were under 40 and 76% were under 50. The corresponding figures for females were 10% under 40 and 63% under 50. Men in top posts were, on average, younger than their female equivalents.

The Salmon Committee suggested that 'it should be possible for some able nurses to look for promotion to Principal Nursing Officer between the ages of 35 and 39, after about 15 years experience of nursing since registration, divided between first line and middle management'.[24] The Committee's only explicit reference to male nurses was in a recommendation that men in general nursing should have equal opportunity with women to be trained and appointed to senior posts.[25] (They had found some 145 men holding senior posts carrying female titles and recommended the abolition of titles distinguished by sex in favour of a unified grading system).

THE NEED FOR REVIEW

The developments outlined above suggest that the time has come for a major reassessment of the role of men in nursing. This was proposed as far back as 1956 by the Nursing Discussion Group at the Ninth World Health Assembly of the World Health Organization.[26] Such a systematic study has unfortunately not materialized. We need to know not only the role which men perform at present but also what contribution they are likely to make to nursing in the future. It could be for instance that men are generally better suited to the responsibilities of administration than women: there is evidence that many female bedside nurses are reluctant to move into managerial positions.[27] But there may well be other areas of nursing in which men could make a distinctive contribution. A good deal of research has been directed towards improving recruitment methods, identifying the causes of wastage of student nurses and improving their training. But, as MacGuire pointed out in a review of the literature on recruitment and wastage,[28] most of this research has concerned female nurses in general hospitals. Up to now very little has been known about the characteristics and attitudes of male recruits to nursing. Even less is known about their progress through training. The most recent figures for the success rate of a representative whole-year cohort of male student nurses refer to 1959.[29]

One of the most important areas concerns the retention of qualified nurses in the profession. The Dan Mason Research Committee discovered that only half of the female nurses who qualified in February 1953 had worked for as much as a year as a staff nurse. By the middle of 1955 24% had already left nursing altogether, mostly for marriage. Nearly half were still working as hospital nurses at that time but the majority did not plan to continue.[30] A further study in 1965 disclosed that only a third of the women who qualified as registered nurses in 1950 and 1959 were still nursing full-time and another 14% part-time. Again, the main problem had been the incompatibility of a nursing career with marriage and a family.[31] In a study of Oxford girls who started training in 1960/61 it was found that only 83% of those who qualified went on to work as staff nurses in the hospital where they trained and only 69% worked as long as six months; to achieve the given complement of staff nurses for a 6 month period, hospitals had to recruit twice that number of students into their training schools.[32] In 1971, the Briggs Committee found that, although only 25% of qualified female nurses and midwives who had left the profession said that they were unlikely to return, the proportion of all female qualified staff who were actually working in the NHS dropped from 71% at ages below 25 to 45% between 25 and 40.[33]

The existing evidence about male nurses indicates that men offer an important alternative to the traditional spinster in all fields of nursing. The Dan Mason Committee found that 82% of men (compared to 44% of women) were still working in hospitals two and a half years after registration in February 1953 and that the majority of them intended to stay. In spite of criticisms of salaries and promotion prospects, marriage is more likely to bind men to a career than to wean them from it, if circumstances are right, and it is probable that most men, once trained, can be counted as permanent additions to the

24

hospital nursing staff. The Salmon Committee noted (without apparently seeing the significance) that only 6% of men above staff nurse level had breaks in their service compared to 28% of corresponding female staff.[34] This stability would seem to enhance men's potential at all levels in the nursing profession.

But clearly the lack of information has limited the possibility of a full appraisal of men's roll in nursing. Dr John Cohen, in his minority report for the post-war working party, pointed to the inadequacy of opinion as a basis for policy on, among other things, the employment of male nurses. The problem was 'sufficiently large and complex to merit a separate enquiry on scientific lines'.[35] The report which follows seeks to support this conclusion and to fill a gap in our knowledge of the nursing profession. Its importance is underlined by the stress placed by the Briggs Committee (who had access to our early findings) on the need to attract more men into nursing.[36]

REFERENCES

1. Department of Health and Social Security (Statistics and Research Division) *Hospital Nursing and Midwifery Staff Tables, at 30th September, 1972.*
2. International Labour Office, *Employment and Conditions of Work of Nurses*, 1960.
3. K. Jones, 'New Light on the Nursing Shortage', *Nursing Times*, 4th August, 1967, p. 1020.
4. Government Social Survey, *Young School Leavers: an Enquiry for the Schools Council*, 1968.
5. D. Vaz, 'High School senior boys' attitudes towards nursing as a career', *Nursing Research*, (1969) Vol. 17, No. 6, p. 533.
6. Royal College of Nursing, *Evidence to the Committee on Nursing*, 1971.
7. P. Morris, *Put Away*, 1969
8. A. McGhie, 'The Role of the Mental Nurse: 3 — Differences in Nursing Attitudes', *Nursing Mirror*, 31st May, 1967, p. 13.
9. A. E. Pavey, *The Story of the Growth of Nursing*, (3rd Ed.), 1951.
10. B. Abel-Smith, *A History of the Nursing Profession*, 1960, p. 4.
11. Ministry of Health, Central Health Services Council, *Psychiatric Nursing: Today and Tomorrow*, 1968.
12. Abel-Smith, *op. cit.*, p. 117
13. Lancet Commission on Nursing, *Final Report*, 1932.
14. Abel-Smith, *op. cit.*, p. 163.
15. Ministry of Health, *Report of the Working Party on the Recruitment and Training of Nurses*, 1948.
16. Department of Health and Social Security (and Ministry of Health), *Hospital Nursing and Midwifery Staff Tables*, (Annually).
17. Figures supplied by the Queen's Institute of District Nursing.
18. J. Rose, 'Bedside Men', *New Society*, 8th August, 1968, pp. 196–7.
19. Ministry of Health and Scottish Home and Health Department, *Report of the Committee on Senior Nursing Staff Structure*, 1966.
20. International Labour Office, *op. cit.*
21. National Board for Prices and Incomes, *Report No. 60: Pay of Nurses and Midwives in the National Health Service*, 1968, para. 132.
22. *Ibid.*, para. 67.
23. Report of the Committee on Senior Nursing Staff Structure, *op. cit.*, Appendix 5.
24. *Ibid.*, para. 9.50.
25. *Ibid.*, para. 9.12.
26. *Chronicle of the World Health Organisation*, Vol. 10, No. 7 (July 1956), p. 213.
27. H. J. Dellar, S. C. Haywood, F. W. Turner, 'Who Wants to be a Manager?', *Nursing Times*, Occasional Papers, 9th January, 1969, pp. 5–7. See also the Report of the Committee on Nursing (Cmnd. 5115, 1972) paras. 524–5.
28. J. M. MacGuire, *Threshold to Nursing*, 1969.
29. General Nursing Council for England and Wales, *Student Nurse Wastage*, 1966.
30. Dan Mason Research Committee. *The Work of Recently Qualified Nurses*, 1956.
31. Dan Mason Research Committee, *Marriage and Nursing*, 1967.
32. J. M. MacGuire, *From Student to Nurse: Part II, Training and Qualification*, Oxford Area Nurse Training Committee, 1966.
33. Report of the Committee on Nursing, *op. cit.*, paras. 65, 412.
34. Report of the Committee on Senior Nursing Staff Structure, Appendix 5.
35. Ministry of Health, Working Party on the Recruitment and Training of Nurses, *Minority Report*, 1948, para. 60.
36. Report of the Committee on Nursing, paras. 96, 414–5, 435.

The broad objectives and overall design of the present survey were agreed after discussions with the Department of Health and Social Security (then the Ministry of Health) in 1966. In summary, the objectives were:

(a) to fill gaps in our information about the educational and career background, motivation, source of recruitment and expectations of male entrants to nurse training;

(b) to find out how men reacted to their training experience, so that consideration could be given to modifying training arrangements in order to suit their needs;

(c) to find out if men experienced special difficulties, not directly connected with their training, which necessitated special arrangements for their reception and welfare;

(d) to identify factors, both individual and institutional, which were associated on the one hand with men's success in training and on the other with premature withdrawal;

(e) to amplify, and test for male entrants, information already collected about nurses in other surveys, particularly about status, career intentions, attitudes to female staff and reactions to training;

(f) as a by-product, to throw up information about this rather unusual group of male employees, particularly in relation to their self-image as men in a women's world.

THE SAMPLE

It was decided to base the survey on a cohort of men who commenced a course of student nurse training at pre-selected nurse training schools during a twelve month period. (We usually refer to the training schools as 'hospitals', which includes groups of hospitals forming a combined school of nursing.) The original plan was to cover hospitals undertaking male nurse training in the Leeds hospital region. It soon became evident that this would yield a sample heavily weighted towards psychiatric training, and containing too few general entrants for effective analysis. The field was therefore enlarged, taking one region at a time and the general hospitals most likely on the basis of recent recruitment figures to have male entrants, until we were reasonably confident of catching 100 general entrants during the calendar year 1968. Psychiatric hospitals were added, with a general view to their representativeness, to yield an expected sample of 250 in mental illness and just over 100 in mental subnormality. Two additional hospitals had to be included towards the end of 1968, when it became apparent that the mental subnormality sample was falling seriously short of expectations. The survey eventually covered entrants to fifty-five training schools in six Regional Hospital Board areas, plus a State Special Hospital and a London teaching hospital. Some balance was maintained between schools in conurbations, urban and rural areas; but it was difficult to achieve a proportional representation of small and isolated hospitals. Details of the hospitals are given in Appendix I.

In the event, the survey population fell short of the target number of students both in general and in mental subnormality training. But it was enriched by the presence of substantial numbers of pupil nurses. We knew that some men were admitted to the two year pupil training,

TABLE 2.1

Survey population compared with overall male recruitment in
England and Wales for 1968
(expected survey population in brackets)

Field of nursing*	No. of hosps.	Survey population			Total male entrants in 1968†			Survey Population as % of total entrants		
		Students	Pupils	Post-reg. students	Students	Pupils	Post-reg. students	Students	Pupils	Post-reg. students
								%	%	%
General	25	79 (100)	43 (10)	61 (100)	577	452	386	13.7	9.5	15.8
Mental Illness	19	201 (250)	34 (16)	6 (43)	1140	264	105	17.6	12.8	5.7
Mental Subnormality	13	92 (110)	17 (2)	9 (7)	380	86	60	24.2	19.7	15.0
Total (expected)	57	372 (460)	94 (28)	76 (150)	2097	802	551	17.7	11.7	13.8

* Students in general hospitals were training for the qualification of State Registered Nurse (SRN), those in mental illness hospitals for that of Registered Mental Nurse (RMN) and in mental subnormality hospitals for the qualification of Registered Nurse of the Mentally Subnormal (RNMS). Pupil nurses were training to become State Enrolled Nurses (SEN).

† Source: Statistics supplied by the General Nursing Council for England and Wales.

but did not set out to cover these entrants as a group, although we were prepared to interview any who appeared at hospitals which we had included on other grounds. As it turned out, the inclusion of pupils not only enabled us to make up a reasonable sample of entrants to each field of nursing, but provided a good deal of material that was of considerable interest in itself. We interviewed 94 pupils in addition to 372 students. We also included post-registration student nurses who were already registered nurses, usually in mental nursing, taking a further training for a second qualification at one of the hospitals in the survey. It was hoped that information about their careers and reactions to training would serve as a point of comparison with the men entering nursing for the first time. There were 76 of these in the final population. The distribution of the survey population is given in Table 2.1. In all, the sample included 16% of all the men who started nurse training in England and Wales in 1968.

METHOD

In other to obtain all the information we sought about these men and to test the findings of other surveys it was decided to use structured and largely pre-coded interview questionnaires. In all, thirteen different versions of the two main questionnaires were needed to cover the circumstances of different types of entrant at various stages of training and withdrawal, and it would be impracticable to reproduce them in full. The initial questionnaire for pre-registration students, which was used more than any other, is reproduced as Appendix II.*

The schedules for the first interview were drafted and piloted after discussion with nurses at local hospitals and with other research workers. Their final form included 69 questions, many of them multiple, and many of them derived from questionnaires used in previous studies. This was to facilitate the comparison of our results with others, with particular reference to studies of female nurses in Oxford published in 1961[1] and 1966[2] and a study of young girls in Mansfield published in 1965[3] and, as it turned out, with surveys carried out for the Briggs Committee in 1970–71.[4]

The use of a standardized questionnaire facilitated the use of outside interviewers. Interviewers (male wherever possible) were recruited from universities and other establishments of higher education as well as one or two from hospital administration. A number of briefings were held before the interviewing began, and full instructions were given to the interviewers.

---

* There were separate versions of the initial and second-stage questionnaires for pupil nurses and post-registration students. In both the wording was varied in questions referring to the specific course or qualification, and, in the case of post-registration students, to their previous training and career. There were separate versions of the second questionnaire for those men who (a) left nursing altogether (b) changed hospital and (c) changed their status from student to pupil or *vice versa.*

The first questionnaire was administered approximately four weeks after the men started in the training school at some time during 1968. The procedure was that hospitals agreed to notify the names of new male entrants in time for an appointment to be made with an interviewer at the desired point in the training programme. (Hospitals also undertook to notify the names and last-known addresses of any men who abandoned their training; apart from that, subsequent contacts were initiated from Hull at the appropriate times.) The hospitals had agreed to allow the men to be interviewed in duty time, usually in the training school itself, to avoid the risk of refusals. Inevitably there were a few gaps – entrants who were missed or who were unwilling to be interviewed. But apart from the two hospitals which were not included in the survey until towards the end of the year, so that we missed two intakes altogether, we managed to interview all but 51 of the starters in the 57 hospitals – a response rate of 91%.

As a result of discussions with the Psychology Department at Hull University concerning suitable intelligence tests, it was decided to use the untimed version of Raven's Progressive Matrices test and the Mill Hill Vocabulary test. The former is a non-verbal test, suitable for overseas as well as English-speaking entrants, giving a measure of intellectual capacity.[5] The latter gives a measure of present attainment and command of the English language.[6]

After consultation with Dr Sybil Eysenck of the Maudsley Institute of Psychiatry, it was also decided to include the PEN, a modified version of the Eysenck Personality Inventory. This personality test had not been published at the time but had been validated and sex norms were available. The PEN, like the two intelligence tests, is self-administered and is also very short, taking no more than ten minutes to complete. All the hospitals that administered the Matrices and Mill Hill tests agreed to include the PEN at the same time, although the latter was not introduced until after the survey had commenced. Otherwise, apart from cases where men refused to take the tests, all three were administered at the first contact. The Mill Hill and Matrices tests were completed by 456 entrants and the personality inventory by 404. 398 men completed all three tests.

During 1968 the second questionnaires were finalized. For most entrants these were administered after completion of the first year in training, to find out about their reactions and to plot any changes in their attitudes over the year. Questionnaires were also prepared for use with men who withdrew from training before the second interview. These might have given up nursing altogether or changed their status, their hospital or both. One or two gave up in the early months and were re-interviewed when they started again later in the year.

Unfortunately, for various reasons we were unable to interview more than 38 of the 132 men who did withdraw from training during the first year. Most of the ones we missed were not traced (by us or by the hospital). We did however interview all except 15 of the 410 who were still in training after a year – a response rate of 96.3%. The details are given in Table 2.2.

TABLE 2.2
Number who did (stayers) or did not (leavers) complete the first year
(number re-interviewed in brackets)

	STAYERS				LEAVERS			
	Students	Pupils	Post-reg.	Total	Students	Pupils	Post-reg.	Total
General	63	34	58	155	16	9	3	28
	(62)	(34)	(54)	(150)	(4)	(2)	(–)	(6)
Mental illness	138	19	5	162	63	15	1	79
	(132)	(18)	(5)	(155)	(20)	(4)	(–)	(24)
MSN	72	14	7	93	20	3	2	25
	(71)	(13)	(6)	(90)	(8)	(–)	(–)	(8)
Total	273	67	70	410	99	27	6	132
	(265)	(65)	(65)	(395)	(32)	(6)	(–)	(38)

Apart from the interviews with the male entrants and the results of the personality and intelligence tests, we also obtained information from the staff of the hospitals and training schools. For each entrant we thus have background information about the hospital where he started training, including its size, staffing and training arrangements, and recent wastage experience. Some of the main features are summarized in Appendix I. Much of the statistical data was taken from regular DHSS returns, supplemented by more qualitative information from an interview with a senior member of the nursing staff.

For each entrant we also obtained a tutor's assessment made at the end of one year's training, along with a record of his absences and the training actually undertaken during that year. For leavers the information covered the reasons for leaving as given to the hospital and training details up to the time of leaving.

Finally, we were fortunate to have an overall assessment of each training school given informally and in confidence by a General Nursing Council Inspector of training schools. The assessment was based on a recent visit by an Inspector and took account of a range of agreed criteria. Schools were allocated to one of three 'grades' with an equal number in each for each field of nursing. The three grades are subsequently referred to as the 'top' 'middle' and 'lower' assessment groups. The award of a 'lower' grading did not imply that the training school was unsatisfactory or failed to meet the standards of the GNC, but it did mean that the Inspectors had a higher opinion of schools in the 'middle' or 'top' grades.

FOLLOW-UP
After the second interviews, which took place throughout 1969, we were not in direct contact with the survey population. Contact was

however maintained with the hospitals in order to check on each man's progress. Forms were sent to the hospitals as men were due for completion of training. In the case of pre-registration student nurses this was normally after three years' training, although concessions were available in recognition of previous spells of uncompleted training and for those who were already enrolled nurses. We knew of these special factors from the first interview schedule. Pupil nurses normally completed training for enrolment after two years. Post-registration students usually took their examinations after eighteen months, although the training period could be as little as twelve months for nurses going from one mental field to another (RMN to RNMS or vice versa). In each case the training period could be extended on account of contingencies such as illness and examination failure. As each individual approached the date on which he was expected to qualify for registration or enrolment, his hospital was asked for details of examination success or failure and subsequent employment. We also obtained definite information about withdrawals at this time. This procedure was repeated when the first inquiry revealed that the man's training had been extended beyond the expected date. In this way, we were able to build up a complete picture of the success and wastage of the original survey population over the whole training period.

The hospitals at which the men completed their training, or to which they moved immediately afterwards, are being contacted again two years after the date of qualification for details of the men's subsequent careers. Some of the follow-ups have already been completed but the final picture will not be available until 1974.

ANALYSIS

The questionnaires used in the survey were largely pre-coded, in that certain responses or pieces of information were allocated a particular 'code', which was simply ringed by the interviewers. These formed the basis of the computer coding which was carried out on all the survey material. The coding for open-ended questions was drawn up after a preliminary analysis of early questionnaires. The data was transferred to punch cards and processed on the Hull University ICT 1905E computer, using the ECXP survey analysis programme which was made available by the University of Essex. The data eventually occupied the greater part of fourteen 80-column cards for each of the 542 cases in the survey population.

The analysis itself was designed to use the basic ECXP operations, i.e. frequency counts and cross-tabulation of different variables. Although the use of the computer involved delays that were frustrating at the time, it has allowed the material to be analysed far more intensively than would otherwise have been possible.

Throughout this report we have used the χ^2 test as a general test of

31

significance, unless otherwise stated. Significance has normally been accepted at the 5% level. Because the sample was not based on a random selection of hospitals we cannot be sure how representative our survey population was of male entrants to nursing as a whole. Within the sample we can be more certain of the significance of differences between various sub-populations. In our findings for the population as a whole we have looked carefully for interrelated trends and consistent patterns which lead cumulatively to the general conclusions we have drawn. With relatively small sub-populations, this has seemed more fruitful than exclusive reliance on statistical tests. The significance of the data has been discussed in the light of previous surveys of female recruits and of other groups of men, and women, in the general population.

REFERENCES

1. J. M. MacGuire, *From Student to Nurse: Part I, the Induction Period*, Oxford Area Nurse Training Committee, 1961.
2. J. M. MacGuire, *From Student to Nurse: Part II, Training and Qualification*, Oxford Area Nurse Training Committee, 1966.
3. D. C. Marsh and A. J. Willcocks *Focus on Nurse Recruitment*, Nuffield Provincial Hospitals Trust, 1965.
4. Report of the Committee on Nursing (Cmnd. 5115, 1972) Appendix I.
5. J. C. Raven *Guide to the Standard Progressive Matrices*, 1960.
6. J. C. Raven, *Guide to using the Mill Hill Vocabulary Scale with the Progressive Matrices Scale*, 1965.

3. CHARACTERISTICS OF MALE RECRUITS

Most of the literature on the recruitment and training of nurses refers almost exclusively to female entrants.[1]

Although men were included in both the GNC's study of student nurses in England and Wales[2] and Scott-Wright's Scottish study,[3] these did not give a clear comprehensive picture of the social and educational backgrounds of male recruits, and gave no information at all about male pupil nurses. Our first questionnaire therefore sought detailed information about backgrounds and pre-nursing careers in order to provide an overall picture of the kind of men who are coming into nursing. Details of the post-registration students are given in the main text for comparison where appropriate, or where a total picture of the survey population is desired. Otherwise figures refer to pre-registration students and pupils. Full details about the post-registration students are given in a separate section.

COUNTRY OF ORIGIN

Both the DHSS and the GNC classify nursing trainees according to their country of birth. We asked the men in our survey population several questions about their cultural origins, including legal nationality, first language, education and upbringing. The nationality question produced the result that 77% of the entrants were British, 6% Irish and 17% of other nationalities. But 25% had spoken a first language other than English and it was clear that nationality as such was not a useful classification.

We then examined all the information about the men's birthplace and upbringing and the interviewer's assessment of skin colour. This led us to a composite classification based on country of origin, being

33

c

the place in which the men had been brought up (and also where most of them had been born). The classification is given in Table 3.1.

TABLE 3.1
The survey population by country of origin and type of training

Country of Origin	Pre-registration students 273 (73%)	Pupils 50 (53%)	Post-registration students 57 (75%)	All 380	% (70%)
British Isles (inc. Eire)					
Commonwealth:					
Mauritius	47	28	2	77	(14%)
India/Pakistan/Ceylon	7	4	1	12	(2%)
Far East[1]	11	1	1	13	(3%)
Africa[2]	14	2	6	22	(4%)
West Indies[3]	7	1	7	15	(3%)
Guyana	4	—	—	4	(1%)
New Zealand	1	—	—	1	(*)
Non-Commonwealth:					
Europe[4]	5	6	1	12	(2%)
Far East[5]	1	—	1	2	(*)
Middle East[6]	2	2	—	4	(1%)
Total Overseas	99 (27%)	44 (47%)	19 (25%)	162	(30%)
Total	372 (100%)	94 (100%)	76 (100%)	542	(100%)

* Less than 0.5%
(1) Malaysia, Hong Kong, Singapore.
(2) Ghana, Sierra Leone, Nigeria, Kenya, Uganda, Zambia, Seychelles.
(3) Jamaica, Trinidad, Barbados, Windward Islands.
(4) Italy, Spain, Portugal, Greece, Holland.
(5) China (Canton).
(6) Jordan, Persia and Morocco.

The most useful distinction for analysis has been between 'British' entrants (i.e. those brought up in the British Isles including Eire, comprising 70% of the survey population) and 'Overseas' (i.e. those from all other countries). All except fourteen of the overseas recruits were non-whites. There were more British entrants in mental illness hospitals and relatively more overseas (particularly Mauritians) in general and mental subnormality. Overseas pupil nurses were concentrated mostly in one or two general hospitals. Four hospitals drew all their 1968 male intake from overseas countries. Just over half the overseas recruits were in hospitals within the Metropolitan Regions.

According to DHSS statistics[4] only 20% of all student and pupil nurses training in English and Welsh hospitals in 1968 had been born overseas. But a recent analysis by the GNC[5] showed that 35% of male students and pupils who started training during 1970/71 were from overseas (compared to only 21% of female students and 29% of female pupils).

At an early stage in the survey, we found that some of the overseas men were somewhat unresponsive and difficult to interview. This applied particularly in the case of Mauritian entrants. For this reason we shortened the questionnaire for subsequent interviews with Mauritian entrants. Where this group were not asked certain questions it will be noted in the text.

34

AGE

The typical female student starts training at the minimum age of 18. Very few wait until they are 21 or over. We expected male entrants to be rather older. But we did not expect the wide variation that we in fact found in starting ages.

Only 22% of the students and 19% of the pupils started at the minimum age of 18. The majority (53% of the students and 67% of the pupils) were over 21 on entry. (Nineteen students, however, were already State Enrolled Nurses). Eight per cent of the students and 17% of the pupils were over thirty and a few were over forty. Students in mental subnormality hospitals tended to be older than the others: 61% started at 21 or over and only 15% at 18 (compared with about a quarter of students entering general or mental illness nursing). More of the British entrants were early starters.

TABLE 3.2

Age at commencement of training

	Students		Pupils	
	British	Overseas	British	Overseas
N = 100%	273	99	50	44
18	29%	7%	32%	5%
19 or 20	28%	19%	12%	16%
21 to 25	27%	50%	18%	45%
over 25	16%	24%	38%	34%

EDUCATION

Altogether, 35% of the male students and pupils completed their full-time education at 14 or 15, 17% at 16 and 48% at 17 or above. Entrants to general training had spent longer in full-time education than the others. There was a considerable difference between British and overseas entrants: 30% of the British students and 18% of the pupils continued in full-time education to 17 or later, compared to 90% of the overseas students and 91% of the pupils: most of the overseas entrants who said they had been receiving full-time education at 18 or over were Mauritian.

There were similar differences in educational attainment (see Table 3.3). Fifty-seven per cent of the total did not have any O-level passes (or equivalent) and another 11% did not satisfy the GNC's normal standard for students of two O-level passes including English. But 32% (34% of the students and 25% of the pupils) did reach the minimum standard, including 17% with five or more O-levels; several had A-levels and three were graduates. The overseas entrants were on the whole better qualified than the British and, in the case of the pupils, perhaps over-qualified: two graduates from overseas started on pupil training, one after being re-graded from student, but had left by the end of the first year.

TABLE 3.3

Educational qualifications

	Students		Pupils	
	British	Overseas	British	Overseas
N = 100%	273	99	44	50
No. of O-level passes or equivalent				
None*	63%	32%	92%	34%
Less than two (or two without English)*	13%	5%	8%	14%
2 – 4 (including 3 or more excluding English)	12%	22%	—	25%
5 or more (including A-levels and degree)	12%	41%	—	27%

* Below normal GNC requirements for entry to student nurse training; there are no formal requirements for pupil training.

In 1968/69, 51% of all entrants to student nurse training possessed GCE qualifications acceptable to the General Nursing Council; in 1970/71 the proportion was 60%.[6] Only 34% of the students in our sample held comparable qualifications. The male pupils on the other hand were better qualified than most of their counterparts. Thirty-five per cent of them had some qualifications (including 25% with qualifications above the minimum standard for student training) compared to 14% of a large sample of mostly female pupils surveyed by the GNC in 1968.[7] It is important to note that 63% of the overseas students and 52% of the overseas pupils had qualifications at or above the minimum standard for student training.

About two-thirds of all the students and about half of all the pupils underwent some sort of training or education after leaving school. Half of each group sat an examination at the end of the course, and nearly all passed it.

When we put together information about the type of school attended by British entrants, their GCE results, age of completing education and age of starting nurse training, a pattern began to emerge. Nearly two-thirds of the British students who entered below the age of 21 had stayed on beyond the minimum school-leaving age, compared to about a third of those who entered at 21 or over. Grammar school entrants had more years of education – only 8% finished at 15 – and the majority (69%) of them entered nursing at 18 to 20. Overall 29% of the British entrants below 21 satisfied the normal educational requirements, compared with 9% of those aged 21 and over. Indeed, three-quarters of those with any formal qualifications at all entered at 20 or below. To put the same point in another way, half of those with GNC minimum entry standards started nurse training within a year of completing their education and two-thirds started within two years.

It was not possible to analyse the overseas recruits' education in the same depth. Nevertheless it was clear that the majority had persisted with their education beyond the normal English school-leaving age in order to obtain their relatively high qualifications. Many of the Mauritians for instance had maintained their studies at home after leaving school. Three-quarters of the overseas men were over 21 when they started nurse training.

MARITAL STATUS

We expected to find that a substantial number of our entrants were married. In fact 82% were single at the time of the first interview, 16% were married and 2% widowed, separated or divorced. (Even among the post-registration students, nearly two-thirds (63%) were single). Among students and pupils, British entrants were more likely to be married (13% students and 20% pupils compared to 11% of the overseas students and 7% of the pupils); but even here, 66% of entrants aged 21 or over were single.

SOCIAL CLASS

Compared with female entrants, fewer of the British men came from middle-class backgrounds and correspondingly more from the Registrar-General's Social Class IV and V (see Table 3.4). Nearly two-thirds of the sample had fathers in manual work, compared with less than half the female students recruited to Scottish non-psychiatric hospitals in 1957–8.[3]

TABLE 3.4

Social class of father's occupation (British)

	Students	Pupils
Excluding unknown or no answer	38	11
N = 100%	235	39
I. Professional occupations	1%	—
II. Intermediate occupations	19%	8%
III. Skilled occupations – non-manual	18%	5%
– manual	37%	69%
IV. Semi-skilled – non-manual	4%	—
– manual	13%	13%
V. Unskilled occupations	8%	5%

EMPLOYMENT EXPERIENCE

Most of the entrants had a gap, averaging between three and five years, between completing school or other full-time education and starting nurse training. The length of the gap varied between students and pupils and between entrants to different fields of nursing. Forty-four per cent of the MSN students had a gap of over five years compared with 30% of general students. Conversely, only a fifth of MSN entrants started training within two years of completing full-time education as against two fifths of general entrants.

TABLE 3.5

Gap between completing full-time education and nurse training

	Students	Pupils
N = 100%	372	94
up to 2 years	30%	31%
between 2 and 5 years	31%	25%
over 5 years	39%	44%

We looked at what British entrants had been doing during this time. Most had been in employment, with an average of three jobs (although about 5% had been in more than ten jobs). Only 3% had no jobs at all. Most (85%) had spent at least a year on one job; 36% of the students and 54% of the pupils had stayed at one job for three years or more. Thirty one per cent of the students and 36% of the pupils had experienced at least one spell of unemployment. About a third had gone into skilled manual occupations on leaving school and another third went into clerical jobs or became shop assistants. Most of the rest took semi-skilled or unskilled manual occupations.

The highest level of skill reached in any job was normally skilled manual (38% of the students and 64% of the pupils) or non-manual (35% of the students and 22% of the pupils). Most of the remainder stayed at the semi-skilled level. For over half, the last job before starting nurse training was semi-skilled manual (which would include work as an auxiliary nurse). One hundred and forty-seven (54%) of the British students and 20 (40%) of the British pupils had at one time held jobs which included some form of training. Only a third, however, had held any previous job for three years or more.

Most of the overseas students and pupils had been recruited in this country and had previously held unskilled manual jobs (including a high-class lift attendant who had worked at Harrods and the Savoy). On the other hand, a number of the nurses recruited in their own countries had been in teaching, government service and other similar non-manual occupations. But many, particularly the Mauritians, had experienced fairly long periods of unemployment in their own countries.

INTELLIGENCE AND PERSONALITY[8]

The Mill Hill and Progressive Matrices tests were administered to 456 men and the Eysenck Personality Inventory (PEN) to 404. (The data are not available for the whole sample because it was not decided to introduce the tests until the survey was already under way.)

Intelligence

Scores on the Mill Hill and the Matrices tests are both expressed in terms of the scores achieved by the general population. It has been suggested that those who come into the bottom quarter of the normal population may be unsuitable for nurse training.[9]

The nurses in our survey scored above average on the Matrices test compared to the general population (see Table 3.6). Scores on the Mill Hill test tended to cluster around the average, only one in six falling below the bottom quartile. It is usually assumed that a lower grading on Mill Hill than on the Matrices indicates undeveloped intellectual capacity. Lack of normal familiarity with the English language also reduces an individual's score on the Mill Hill test. It has therefore been suggested that the Mill Hill test is not appropriate for overseas applicants; others have suggested that non-British subjects may also be at a disadvantage in the Matrices test.[10] The overseas men in our sample did in fact register lower scores than the British, particularly on the Mill Hill, in spite of having better educational qualifications.

There were no important differences between entrants to general and psychiatric training. The lowest groups, as we might expect, included disproportionately more of those undertaking the shorter and more practical pupil nurse training. But both categories of entrants were well represented in the higher ranges.

TABLE 3.6

Raven's Progressive Matrices test and Mill Hill Vocabulary test
Distribution of scores for male student and pupil nurses (including post-registration students), by country of origin

| | | RPMT | | MHVT | |
		British	Overseas	British	Overseas
N = 100%		321	135	321	135
	% in normal population				
Grade 1	5%	15%	10%	2%	—
Grade 2	20%	41%	18%	19%	3%
Grade 3	50%	38%	47%	73%	53%
Grade 4	20%	6%	18%	6%	42%
Grade 5	5%	*	7%	—	2%

* Less than 0.5%

39

Personality

The PEN test is designed to estimate degrees of psychoticism, neuroticism and extraversion-introversion. It also includes a 'lie' scale.

(i) Psychoticism

Individuals who score high on the psychoticism (P) scale can be expected to dislike people, to be likely to go out of their way to cause trouble but, on the other hand, to be relatively 'cold-blooded' i.e. possibly better equipped to keep cool in circumstances that might cause stress in more sensitive people.

The male nurses in our sample were slightly (but not significantly)* more psychotic than the normal population. Overseas entrants had significantly higher P scores than the British entrants (see Table 3.7).

(ii) Extraversion

Those who score high on extraversion are sociable people, often impulsive, with relatively high activity drives which could, in extreme cases, lead to a slapdash approach to responsibility. On the other hand, high extraversion should be useful for a nurse in making it easier for her to deal with people.

Our sample of male nurse trainees were significantly (p<.01) more extraverted than the normal population and also in comparison with female entrants to nursing.

(iii) Neuroticism

One might expect successful nurses to be less neurotic than the normal population. Highly neurotic people would tend to be irritable with patients and staff and unable to stand the strain of nursing. Those who were very neurotic would probably drop out. There would therefore be good reasons for suspecting the suitability for nursing of people with a high N score.

The male nurses were significantly (p<.01) less neurotic than the normal population. Their low N scores are particularly significant in nursing terms and it was interesting to note that the post-registration students had an even lower average N score (mean 5.28, S.D. 3.77) than the others. (It is therefore rather surprising that the high N-scores shown in table 3.7 have been found in groups of female student nurses).

(iv) 'Lie' Score

Part of the PEN Inventory is designed to test whether respondents are giving truthful answers to other questions. In particular, a high 'lie' score tends to be associated in some cases with unexpectedly low N scores. High L scores also tend to be registered by people who feel themselves to be outsiders, including foreigners.

* A *t* test of significance was used for all differences between means.

TABLE 3.7

Psychoticism, Extraversion, Neuroticism and 'Lying'

Scores of the male nurse sample and other groups in the general population

	P Mean	P S.D.	E Mean	E S.D.	N Mean	N S.D.	L Mean	L S.D.	N
All male student and pupil nurses in survey	2.56	2.36	13.77	3.41	6.79	3.96	5.76	4.02	404
British students and pupils	2.02	2.05	13.64	3.63	6.86	4.00	4.11	2.96	274
Overseas students and pupils	3.84	2.22	13.97	2.91	6.77	3.95	9.18	3.74	130
Other male groups									
Students	2.39	2.55	13.17	3.91	9.38	4.43			700
Age 20–29	2.11	2.75	12.28	4.05	7.72	4.25	†		124
General population	2.50	2.71	12.75	4.12	7.33	4.37	4.56	2.95	1012
Female groups									
Student nurses*	†		12.57	4.31	11.50	4.49	†		1005
Students	1.68	1.82	12.72	3.41	10.52	3.69	†		700
Age 20–29	1.41	1.97	12.15	3.56	8.52	4.17	†		68
General population	2.02	2.22	12.36	3.68	8.64	4.35	†		1320

* Scores on the E.P.I.   † Data not available.

Source: Eysenck, S. B. G. and Eysenck, H. J.: 'Scores on Three Personality Variables as a Function of Age, Sex and Social Class', *British Journal of Social and Clinical Psychology* (1969), 8, pp. 69–76.

The L scores of the male nurses were significantly higher (p=.01) than the normal population. But according to Eysenck[11] this does not necessarily provide much evidence of lying, since the mean is within one quarter of the standard deviation for the control group. There was a negative correlation (0.26) between L and N scores, which suggested a moderate motivation to 'fake good'. Overseas students scored exceptionally high on the L scale particularly those from Mauritius (a mean of 10.38 compared to 4.11 for British entrants) which ties in with the expectation that outsiders would be inclined to search for socially acceptable answers to a questionnaire and justifies our decision to exclude Mauritians from part of the first questionnaire. (On the other hand, the N scores of the Mauritians were only slightly lower than those of the other entrants and there were no significant differences on P and E scores).

POST-REGISTRATION STUDENTS

Initial Training

Fifty-nine (78%) of the 76 post-registration students had initially qualified as RMN, ten (13%) RMNS and five (7%) SRN. Another two had taken integrated courses leading to both the RMN and RNMS qualifications. Two of the RMNs had later also qualified as SRN.

All the students had been trained in British or Irish hospitals, although three men (all Africans) also held nursing qualifications from other countries. (Altogether 31 (41%) of the students had been born and brought up abroad, twelve of them in Ireland).

At the start of their first training the average age of the post-registration students had been 21 (slightly lower than the average starting age among the pre-registration students in our survey population). The majority had taken the normal three years to complete their first training. However 19 (25%) of them had taken more than three years and three months including three who had taken over four years.

Field Changes

Table 3.8 gives details of field of nursing for the men's previous and post-registration training.

Only 26 (34%) of the men had been seconded for further training by their parent hospitals on full pay. Twenty were from mental illness hospitals, two from general and four from MSN hospitals. The remainder had made their own arrangements, which normally involved a loss of pay during training.

Career after First Qualification

At the time they started their post-registration training in 1968 the

42

TABLE 3.8

Post-registration students: field of training by previous nursing field

| n = 76 | Post-registration training | | | |
	General	Mental illness	MSN	Total
General	—	3	2	5
Mental Illness	52	—	5	57
MSN	7	3	—	10
Mental Illness and General	—	—	2	2
Mental Illness and MSN	2	—	—	2
Total	61	6	9	76

average age of the students was 26, the youngest being 21 and the oldest 37. After gaining their first qualification 51% of the students had spent less than a year nursing before starting on their second training: over a third (36%) had completed their initial training less than six months previously and four men had in fact gone straight on without a break. Of the remainder, over half (26% of the total) had been nursing for more than two years since qualification, including seven men with five or more years' service.

During this time the great majority (82%) of the students had worked as staff nurses in the hospitals where they had trained, three-quarters of them for less than two years. Only one man had stayed in the same hospital and been promoted to Charge Nurse. (He already held the dual RMN/RNMS qualification). The rest, apart from the four students who had gone straight from first to second training, had changed hospitals at some time. Three men had moved in order to train for SRN and two had been successful. Both had subsequently been promoted to Charge Nurse. Of the other eight men who had moved, six had remained as staff nurses but one had been promoted to Deputy Charge Nurse and the other to Charge Nurse.

SUMMARY

Our survey population was thus fairly heterogeneous, and more varied than the normal cohort of female entrants to nurse training. Four-fifths were over the minimum age of 18, and the majority were over 21. A third had left school at 14 or 15. Less than half had any educational qualifications at all, and two thirds did not meet the GNC requirements. The best-qualified groups educationally were those who started nurse training at 18, those training in general hospitals, and those born and brought up outside the British Isles, who constituted nearly a third of the male intake to the hospitals in the survey.

Some of the overseas entrants, including two graduates, seemed over-qualified for the pupil training schemes on which we found them.

In terms of intelligence test scores, the men included a fair number of the highest ability. Their personality profiles suggested that they were on the whole suited to nursing and rather more so than comparable groups of female entrants. They were significantly more extraverted and less neurotic than the normal population, and did not exhibit the characteristic 'instability syndrome' of students – a combination of high extraversion and high neuroticism. In particular they registered less neuroticism than comparable groups of female student nurses.

REFERENCES

1. J. M. MacGuire, *Threshold to Nursing*, 1969.
2. General Nursing Council for England and Wales, *Student Nurse Wastage*, 1966.
3. M. Scott-Wright, *Student Nurses in Scotland: Characteristics of Success and Failure*, Scottish Home and Health Department, 1968.
4. Department of Health and Social Security (Statistics and Research Division), *Overseas born student and pupil nurses and pupil midwives in training in National Health Service Hospitals in England and Wales*, at 31st December, 1968.
5. Figures supplied by the General Nursing Council Research Unit.
6. General Nursing Council, *Annual Reports*.
7. A. Singh, 'The Predictive Value of Cognitive Tests for Selection of Pupil Nurses', *Nursing Times* Occasional Papers, June 8, 1972, pp. 89–92.
8. For a more complete discussion of the material summarised here, see 'Personality and Intelligence Characteristics of Male Nurses', *International Journal of Nursing Studies*, Vol. 9, pp. 167–177, 1972.
9. P. Pearson 'Selection at the Pre-Nursing Stage', *Nursing Times*, February 9, 1968, pp. 188–189.
10. T. G. Crookes and J. C. French 'Intelligence and Wastage of Student Mental Nurses', *Occupational Psychology* (1961), Vol. 35, pp. 149–154.
11. H. J. Eysenck, 'Relation between Intelligence and Personality', *Perceptual and Motor Skills* (1971) Vol. 32, pp. 637–638.

4. THE CHOICE OF NURSING

GENERAL INTRODUCTION

Other research on young workers has shown that home and educational background influences boys' job aspirations, their attitudes to the satisfactions of work and also the means by which they seek and obtain a job.[1, 2, 3, 4, 5]

Boys from white-collar homes who leave grammar schools at 16+ with GCE qualifications are more likely than secondary modern leavers to make a positive choice of employment (usually non-manual) and to receive skilled help in finding it. At the other end of the continuum, 15 year-old secondary modern leavers from manual backgrounds, with no educational qualifications, are likely to receive haphazard, ill-informed advice on careers and to enter manual employment out of which there is little chance of movement. Attainment at school tends to be associated both with the motivation to take, and with success in, further education, which thus tends to reinforce earlier education and not compensate for it.

Attitudes to work itself can be distinguished according to the importance of intrinsic and extrinsic rewards. At one extreme is the boy in a manual occupation who looks to his job for purely extrinsic satisfactions (pay, security, good workmates, working hours and conditions) and at the other the non-manual boy who seeks intrinsic satisfactions (interesting work, ability to make decisions, tasks matching his abilities, responsibility and pride in his work). Promotion prospects can be regarded as intrinsic or extrinsic, according to whether they are seen as the means for achieving a higher position and greater responsibility (and hence intrinsic satisfaction) or merely for getting more money.

Occupations may be chosen according to one set of motives and actual jobs according to another set. Alternatively (as possibly with nursing) a choice based on mainly intrinsic factors may be rationalized or legitimized to one's peers by reference to extrinsic factors.

The final choice of job is influenced again by home and educational background in the extent and nature of advice which is offered and taken. It may be 'inner directed' i.e. based on the boy's abilities and inclinations; or it may be directed by family and neighbourhood traditions; or it may be 'other directed' with reference to outside influences including the status of the job in the community. According to one study,[1] tradition still accounts for about a fifth of the job choices of secondary modern boys. According to another,[2] personal contacts are the most important single means through which 15 year old school leavers find a particular job.

Nursing is not a frequent choice for boys at the time they leave school. A study of children nearing school-leaving age in the south of England in 1956 discovered only one boy out of 702 who wanted to become a nurse, compared with 78 out of 600 girls (13%).[1] A larger and more representative study for the Schools Council ten years later found between 2% and 5% (according to prospective school leaving age) of schoolgirls intending to enter the nursing and medical ancillary professions, and between 3% and 8% of young women aged 19 or 20 who had actually done so. But there were no candidates at all among comparable samples of schoolboys and young men.[2] It seems likely, therefore, that the men who do choose nursing are untypical in some ways, e.g. by having a close family connection with the profession or through having found themselves in medical units in the Forces. Another possibility is that many of the older entrants have turned to nursing after a false start elsewhere, and are attracted either by the opportunity to give service or by the chance to obtain the status and security of a recognized qualification.

We have therefore tried to identify the channels through which the male pre-registration student and pupil nurses came into nursing and the various factors which influenced their choice, including previous contact with nursing. As far as possible, their career-choice processes are compared with those of other young men and women in Britain. For this reason, and because different factors are likely to be operating in different cultural contexts, British and overseas entrants are considered separately in the various sections in this chapter.

PREVIOUS CONTACTS WITH NURSING: BRITISH ENTRANTS

Family Contacts

Although not large, the proportion of men with fathers who had actually worked in a hospital was greater than one would expect in an average cross-section of the population. Seven per cent of the

46

students and 4% of the pupils had fathers who had nursed. A further 4% of the students' fathers and 6% of the pupils' had had non-nursing jobs in hospital.

Far more of the entrants had a hospital connection through their mother. Twenty per cent of the students and 14% of the pupils had mothers who were or had been nurses. An additional 8% of the students' mothers and 10% of the pupils' had worked in non-nursing jobs in hospital. Overall, a third of the general entrants had mothers who had worked in a hospital but only a fifth of those starting on mental subnormality training. The distribution of father contacts, however, was constant between fields.

In addition, 12% of the students and 14% of the pupils had brothers or sisters who had nursed. The number of siblings with non-nursing jobs in hospital was insignificant.

Altogether, a third of the students and pupils had at least one member of the immediate family who was or had been a nurse. Nearly a third of these had nursed in the hospital where the men were training. Over two-fifths had a similar family contact with some hospital job. These family contact rates are much higher than those found among girls in their upper teens who were not in nursing (and whose degree of contact is therefore likely to be representative of both sexes in the general population).[6, 7] But they are equalled or surpassed by girls actually in nursing: in one survey those who had relatives in hospital jobs comprised 80% of the nurses, 35% of girls interested in nursing and 20% of other girls.[6] So it looks as if family contacts are important for the recruitment of nurses of both sexes, contact through a nursing parent being particularly important for men.

Other research has suggested that the *attitude* of relatives is an important influence in the decision to take up nursing. In our study, well over half the mothers, but rather less than half the fathers, were said to have been 'keen' or 'very keen' on their sons taking up nursing. (In Scott-Wright's study of student nurses in Scotland[8] three-quarters of the nurses said their parents had favoured their career choice and parental encouragement also seemed important for success in training). Table 4.1 shows that parents who had worked in hospitals themselves were more favourable than others. Parents who had actually been nurses showed even more favourable attitudes: 87% of mothers and 72% of fathers who had nursed were 'very keen' or 'quite keen'.

Parental contact was also associated with age of entry. Twenty-five per cent of those who started training under 21 had mothers who had nursed as against 12% of the others. There were similar, but less striking, differences for the proportion with fathers and/or siblings in nursing who entered at different ages. Overall, 70% of entrants whose mothers had nursed, and 62% of those whose fathers or siblings had nursed, started training before the age of 21 compared with 54% of all entrants.

TABLE 4.1
Parents' attitudes to respondent (students and pupils) taking up nursing

| | Mother | | Father | |
	Worked in hospital	Not worked	Worked in hospital	Not worked
N = 100%	88	235	38	285
Very keen	53%	21%	47%	15%
Quite keen	26%	29%	21%	24%
Indifferent	8%	20%	10%	26%
Not very keen	7%	13%	10%	6%
Not at all keen	—	8%	3%	6%
Parent dead/not seen for many years	6%	9%	9%	23%

Only a third of our respondents were able to give any answer to a question about their parents' ambitions for them on leaving school and only a tiny proportion of these (4% of students) related to nursing. But 14% gave as a reason for taking up nursing the fact that a parent or a relative was a nurse. Only another 4% of students and 2% of pupils mentioned knowing someone other than a parent or relative in this context.

Other contacts

Two thirds of the men in our survey had known someone in nursing, apart from parents and siblings. (Other surveys suggest that a third to two-fifths of girls in the general population have a close friend who is a nurse.)[6, 7] Indeed, only a quarter had known nobody, family or otherwise, who had nursed at one time or another. When asked whether these contacts had encouraged or discouraged them, most of the men gave neutral or mixed answers but the general attitude seemed to be one of encouragement. Sixteen per cent of general entrants (but only 6% of the others) remembered someone advising them against nursing because it had low status, stigma, or was 'not a man's job'.

Nineteen per cent of the students and 26% of the pupils had belonged to a nursing organization (mostly the St John's Ambulance Brigade) before taking up nursing. Higher attachment rates have been found among girls – even those who do not become nurses; but we would guess that this is a fairly high rate for men. About two-thirds (rising to 85% of the general entrants) had been in hospital as a patient.

Only 15% said that they had listened to careers talks at school on nursing. (The proportion of teenage girls, not in nursing, who remember such a talk tends to vary between a third and 45%.)[6] Most of the men who had listened to such talks did not consider them important in creating an image of the profession. Nor was much importance credited to the representation of nursing in plays, films and novels. Less than a quarter, in fact, had read nursing novels. About half had read nursing leaflets or a nursing weekly and a slight majority of these agreed that they contained important information.

None of these impersonal sources of contact was said to have been as important in building up an image of nursing as work-experience in a hospital or talking with people who were connected with nursing – which three-quarters of the students and rather more of the pupils had done.

Employment related to nursing

Over 70% of the students and three-quarters of the pupils (but only 54% of general trainees) had some earlier experience of hospital work. In most cases this experience was gained as a cadet, pre-student nurse, or nursing auxiliary, often in a job of less than six months duration immediately before taking up nurse training. A handful had been employed as orderlies, clearly as fill-in jobs. Over a third of the students had been in cadet or other pre-nursing schemes, some of them for the whole time since leaving school. Ten (4%) of the students had already qualified as State Enrolled Nurses. A further 15%, and 4% of the pupils, had made previous attempts at nurse training.

These findings can be compared with those from other surveys relating to girls taking up nursing. Thus 79% of a cohort of girls starting training in Oxford hospitals took a paid job before starting nurse training, 60% of them for more than two years, but half said it was only a 'fill-in'. Fifty-seven per cent of them worked in a hospital.[9] Similarly, half of a group of non-psychiatric nurse starters in Scotland had held a previous nursing job and 40% had no job outside nursing. Seventeen per cent, however, had gained some experience on pre-nursing courses and another 19% as orderlies or auxiliaries.[8] A third of the 36 men in that study had previous hospital experience, three having made earlier attempts at student training. For this small group of men, experience of manual work correlated with successful completion of nurse training. An unpublished study of 53 hospitals by the Sheffield Regional Hospital Board discovered that 46% of the student entry (25% in mental hospitals) had previously been cadets.[10] Twenty per cent of the student nurses and 17% of the pupils in the Briggs Committee survey had taken a pre-nursing course; 22% and 14% had been cadets.[11]

Only four students and one pupil (with three post-registration students) had experience of nursing duties in HM Forces, which seems therefore to have lost whatever importance it once had as a source of recruitment of male nurses. (A recent study of qualified male nurses[12] discovered that 31% had started nursing in HM Forces).

PREVIOUS CONTACTS : OVERSEAS ENTRANTS

As with the British entrants, many of the overseas recruits had

49

contacts with other nurses. The majority had known someone who was a nurse, and about a fifth had a nursing parent or sibling. Nine of the students were already State Enrolled Nurses and a further seven (plus three pupils) had a history of discontinued training. Just over half the other students and pupils had worked as assistant or auxiliary nurses in this country before starting their training.

THE DECISION TO NURSE: BRITISH ENTRANTS

About half the girls who are interested in nursing seem to start considering it by the time they are 12 or 13.[6, 7, 8] By contrast, less than one in eight of the men in our sample first considered nursing before they were 15. A majority had not considered it until *after* the minimum age of entry (see Table 4.2).

But there were important differences between fields. Fifty-nine per cent of the entrants to general training said they had considered nursing before the minimum age, compared to 43% of those in hospitals for the mentally ill and 39% in mental subnormality. Almost a third of the mental subnormality entrants had not considered nursing until they were over 21, a point at which the majority of female students are nearly at the end of their training. Only 9% of general entrants became interested so late.

At the time they left school a third of the students and a quarter of the pupils had ambitions for other administrative, professional and technical occupations. Only 40 students and 8 pupils (15% of the British entrants) intended to become nurses. A further 20 (6%) left

TABLE 4.2

Commitment to nursing by age of starting training

	Age started training					Total =
	18	19	20	21–25	26+	100%
Age nursing first considered:*						
Under 15	47%	19%	14%	14%	6%	36
15–17	59%	10%	8%	18%	5%	109
18 and over	7%	15%	14%	32%	32%	173
Time since making definite decision to nurse:†						
Over 2 years	35%	7%	7%	32%	18%	71
1–2 years	53%	12%	8%	13%	14%	51
6–12 months	24%	17%	15%	23%	21%	82
Under 6 months	18%	17%	14%	29%	22%	116
Ambitions on leaving school:						
Nursing	60%	15%	10%	10%	4%	48
'Frustrated' – non-nursing	27%	18%	7%	28%	20%	96
Others, including Don't know, etc.	21%	11%	18%	25%	25%	179
All students	29%	16%	12%	27%	16%	273
All pupils	32%	4%	8%	18%	38%	50

* 5 couldn't recall

† 3 couldn't recall

school with ambitions to work in a field related to nursing, mostly medicine, but also e.g. remedial gymnastics, therapeutic art and dentistry. Eighty-four (26%) did not know or remember their job ambitions and most of the remaining 38% had fairly straightforward plans for entering various occupations.

Roughly, then, a third of those who came into nursing had left school with the definite intention of doing something else, a quarter had no particular ambitions and less than a sixth were thinking of nursing at that time. Rather more of the latter group were found in general hospitals and rather more of those without clear career intentions in psychiatric hospitals. Comparing the whole population with what we know about female entrants, it is evident that for men nursing is much more likely to be a late choice, or an alternative to which they turn after failing to achieve their first ambitions. We found that 30% of all the entrants (77 students and 19 pupils) had been prevented from pursuing their original ambitions either through lack of qualifications for a professional job, or through parental opposition or more simply because there were no local opportunities for a particular career, or occupation. In the event only 12% went into jobs similar in type to those they had wanted, and these were mostly skilled manual jobs or jobs in service industries. At least a fifth went straight into semi-skilled or unskilled work which none had originally wanted. (For comparison, 71% of the girls in the Scottish survey had made nursing their first choice of career. In MacGuire's Oxford study only half the girls starting general training had seriously considered any alternative to nursing, usually teaching.)

The Schools Council survey provides some comparable material for a representative group of school leavers. At school leaving age, over half the boys due to leave at 15 expected manual jobs in manufacturing or engineering. Very few of these aimed at professional or semi-professional jobs. Eight per cent were thinking of uniformed employment in the police, forces, etc., but none of hospital work. About a fifth of the 16 year old and half the 17 year old leavers, however, were aiming at professional and semi-professional employment, although many who had left were disappointed and found themselves in offices. The authors of the survey commented that aspirations tend to shift from manual to professional-type occupations as boys stay longer at school. Two-thirds of the boys still at school hoped for an apprenticeship; and half those who had left school managed to secure one. Those who secured apprenticeships were more stable in subsequent employment.[2]

To sum up this part of the material, the younger British men in our sample had a broadly similar work experience to their female opposite numbers before starting to train as a nurse. They were also more likely than the older entrants to have been at a grammar school, had higher educational attainments, had first considered nursing at an earlier age and were more likely to have definitely decided to nurse a year or

51

more before starting their training. They were more likely to have had a father or mother who was a nurse. The older men came in by a longer route, and their experience on the way was more similar to that of the less successful half of 15 year old school leavers, those who do not get apprenticeships. On the whole they had slightly less family contact with nursing, had a greater variety of non-nursing jobs and in most cases had made a definite decision to nurse less than a year, or in many cases less than six months, before starting nursing. One unusual feature of our sample is perhaps the proportion who left school with ambitions, unrealistic in terms of their educational background, for professional training.

THE DECISION TO NURSE: OVERSEAS ENTRANTS

The pattern for overseas entrants is more confused and more factors seem to be involved. In general they appeared to have considered nursing at a later age than British entrants – two-thirds had been over 18 when they had first considered nursing – but to have taken longer between reaching a definite decision and starting to train. Over 60% had definitely decided over a year before and 38% two years or more before they commenced training. Seventeen per cent had not worked at all before nursing. Most of the others had had jobs in this country, over half of them including spells as nursing assistants or auxiliaries, prior to being accepted as student or pupil nurses. Their career paths suggested that a large proportion of overseas recruits do not originally come to Britain with the intention of training as nurses. (The DHSS statistics[13] show that nearly half the overseas-born student and pupil nurses in training in 1968 were recruited in this country).

MOTIVATION: BRITISH ENTRANTS

To test their general attitudes to training and a career, we asked the men whether they agreed or disagreed with three statements: –

(a) 'A long period of training in a job is a waste of time'. The majority of entrants (84% of students and 62% of pupils) disagreed. Grammar school boys were most likely to disagree.

(b) 'Money is the most important thing about a job'. As expected, the majority (87% and 84%) disagreed with this statement. Those who did agree were rather more likely to withdraw from training in the first twelve months.

(c) 'Few people work night shifts if there is other work available'.

This statement was included to test the belief that awkward hours were less of a disincentive for boys than for girls. Fifty-eight per cent of the male students and 78% of the pupils agreed with it, grammar school boys being rather less likely to agree than ex-secondary modern school boys. This is very similar to the answers in the Mansfield and

Huddersfield studies[6,7] of girls in the general population, two thirds of whom agreed with the statement. It therefore seems unlikely that male entrants are unusually indifferent to the pattern of hours they have to work.

Reasons for taking up nursing

Respondents were asked to say how important each of thirteen possible reasons for taking up nursing had been to them in making their own decisions. Possible answers included five degrees of importance and 'didn't consider it'. Table 4.3 shows (a) the percentage who did *not* consider each factor and (b) the average rating that the others gave it on a scale in which 5 = very important indeed, 4 = very important, 3 = important, 2 = not very important and 1 = not at all important.

The factors are arranged roughly in order of importance, which differed slightly for students and pupils, and not in the order in which they were put.

TABLE 4.3

Factors in the Decision to Nurse

	% who did not consider at all		Average rating given by those who did consider it	
	Students	*Pupils*	*Students*	*Pupils*
The opportunity to help other people	1%	—	4.0	4.4
The fact that a nurse is dealing with people rather than things	1%	2%	4.1	4.3
The chance to learn something new	4%	6%	3.7	3.8
The chance to study while working and learning	5%	—	3.5	3.7
Good prospects of promotion	5%	8%	3.4	3.2
Working with people with similar interests	9%	—	3.3	3.7
The fact that a nurse is paid while he is being trained	9%	4%	3.1	3.4
The fact that a nurse need never be out of a job once qualified	13%	8%	3.8	3.9
The fact that you knew someone who had been a nurse	26%	24%	2.4	2.8
The opportunity to work near home	26%	24%	2.0	2.5
The fact that you felt like a change	27%	20%	2.5	2.6
The opportunity to work away from home	41%	42%	2.3	2.1
The sports and recreation facilities	43%	48%	2.2	2.2

Intrinsic aspects of nursing such as helping, working with people and learning are given far more weight than the extrinsic factors of pay, promotion, security and companionship. The results are consistent with surveys of girls' motivation to nurse. Ninety-five per cent of Oxford student nurses rated 'the opportunity to help others' as important or very important; 86% gave equivalent ratings to 'working with people', 63% to security after training and only 28% to pay while training.

The answers were compared for entrants who started training above and below the age of 21. The over 21s gave more importance to the chance to learn something new, the chance to study and the fact that a nurse is paid while training.

Spontaneous answers to an earlier open question about the main reasons for taking up nursing were consistent with the more structured one. About half the men mentioned the intrinsic interest and satisfactions of nursing – particularly those in mental subnormality training. A third of the students and half the pupils gave vocational answers, including the opportunity to help other people; this came particularly strongly from entrants to general training and from those who had considered nursing at an early age. In addition, 14% of the students and 20% of the pupils mentioned the desire to do something worthwhile. One student in five (but rather fewer pupils) mentioned the promotion and career prospects in nursing, and one in six mentioned security; but only 4% specifically mentioned qualifications and the opportunity to study. Entrants to the psychiatric fields (who tended to be older) mentioned career and job-security factors more frequently.

Others gave more circumstantial reasons for their decisions. Over a fifth mentioned various contacts they had had as patients or through relatives and friends who were patients or nurses. Less than a tenth mentioned negative factors ('out of work', 'needed a job') but this rose to 16% in the mental subnormality field. On the other hand, 59% of MSN entrants (compared to less than half those in the other fields) mentioned the intrinsic rewards and satisfactions of the work.

Singh[14] has questioned the validity of the humanitarian motives often given for entering nursing.* We found in our survey that those with high 'lie' scores on the personality inventory were particularly likely to say that they had taken up nursing with the intention of helping people or working with people with similar interests. We must therefore be careful about taking these altruistic statements at their face value: there may have been a tendency to give the interviewer the expected response. But we also formed the impression that many of the men in our survey did have a strong sense of vocation (see below).

Attractive and unattractive features of nursing

No career offers undiluted advantages. We tried to find out which aspects of nursing the men saw as encouraging or discouraging both for men in general and for themselves.

We asked each respondent why he thought more men did not take up nursing. This question was repeated at the second interview, after a year in training. In both interviews, poor pay and the fact that nursing

---

* 'To be dealing with people rather than things', 'opportunities to help other people', 'the opportunity to live and work with people', 'interest in nursing', 'work of service to the community'. Over four-fifths of his sample of female students gave all of these as important or very important in their decision to enter the nursing profession.

was thought of as a woman's job received most mentions. A substantial minority said it was because male nurses were thought to be effeminate and also because of the lack of publicity for nursing as a man's job.

In another question on this subject, the interviewers went through a list of various aspects of nursing asking whether each would be more likely to encourage or discourage men in general from taking up nursing, and also whether any of the factors had encouraged or discouraged the respondent when he was thinking of taking up nursing. The most encouraging aspects of nursing were promotion prospects, holidays and social status. The most discouraging were pay and awkward hours, as distinct from the total number of hours worked. It emerged that a good number of the respondents had been encouraged by the discipline and study involved in nursing, which they thought likely to discourage men in general, and that they were also less put off by the hours and the pay. It is clear that many people, both men and women, enter nursing in spite of misgivings about the pay and hours. Nearly half the men in our sample were earning less as a nurse than in a previous non-nursing job, and a fifth thought they would still be earning less as a nurse in ten years time. We do not know how many other men are put off by these factors. But the entrants whom we interviewed were generally agreed that pay and hours *would* discourage other people.

MOTIVATION: OVERSEAS ENTRANTS

On the question of motivation it was noticeable that the overseas men in general were less forthcoming than the British. The majority gave reasons connected with helping people, doing a rewarding job and other humanitarian motives. Only eight men specifically said they had decided to nurse so that they could come to England. (A survey carried out by PEP in 1971, however, found immigrant nurses and midwives ready to admit that the opportunity to come to Britain was as much a motivating force as the desire to become a nurse or midwife.)[15]

Attractive and unattractive features of nursing

As with the questions about motivation, overseas students and pupils were less forthcoming than the British about the features of nursing that they found attractive or unattractive. They had however been noticeably less discouraged by the pay, by the study they would have to do and by aspects of hospital life such as the discipline. In fact they claimed to have been particularly encouraged by traditional male deterrents such as the fact that most nurses are women.

CHOICE OF FIELD AND HOSPITAL: BRITISH ENTRANTS

Towards the end of the interview, we asked why entrants had

chosen to take up their particular field of nursing. Table 4.4 summarizes the answers from all the British entrants to each type of nursing.

TABLE 4.4

Reasons for choosing a particular field of nursing

(All mentions were coded)	General	Percentage mentioning Mental illness	MSN
N = 100%	67	187	69
Intrinsic interest of the work (challenge; more satisfying; interest in psychology)	24%	61%	43%
Career/promotion prospects	19%	7%	6%
Pay	1%	14%	6%
More of a man's world	—	6%	—
Not accepted by other type of hospital (inc. preferred other type but doubtful of acceptance)	—	4%	6%
Other reasons	27%	12%	10%
Did not make a positive choice	31%	13%	30%

These answers show a high proportion of intrinsic reasons from those starting in mental illness (a result at variance with the Briggs Committee findings)[16] and a surprisingly high percentage of negative or neutral replies from both MSN and general entrants. It is possible, of course, that many of the latter never seriously considered going into another field. Promotion prospects were important as an incentive only for those choosing general training, while the psychiatric pay lead was pulling slightly in the opposite direction.

Table 4.5 summarizes the replies to an open question about how the entrants came to apply to a particular hospital. (A fifth had applied to other hospitals for training and just under half of these had actually been offered places).

TABLE 4.5

Reasons for choosing hospital

(All mentions were coded)	General	Mental illness	MSN
N = 100%	67	187	69
Knew someone nursing there	7%	22%	26%
Local knowledge or reputation of hospital	16%	5%	7%
Had worked there previously	7%	2%	3%
Suggested by Employment Exchange/ Youth Employment Officer	4%	9%	6%
Recommended by nursing or hospital authority	25%	7%	4%
Recommended by relative/friend/school	9%	13%	14%
Saw advertisement in local paper	15%	21%	25%
Saw advertisement in nursing press	4%	3%	—
Only hospital of its kind in the area	24%	25%	17%
Others	4%	4%	3%

Most of the answers referred to extraneous factors – personal contacts, seeing an advertisement, or the lack of choice. Only among the general entrants were there many references to reputation and informed recommendation. Personal contacts had played some part and were mentioned by about a quarter of entrants to the psychiatric fields. (One entrant in three had a nurse in his immediate family).

CHOICE OF HOSPITAL: OVERSEAS ENTRANTS

Some hospitals told us that they maintained official recruiting contacts in various overseas countries. But on the whole more of the overseas than the British entrants based their choice of hospital on informal sources and few of them mentioned formal channels of recruitment, such as their country's High Commission. A quarter of the men said they had come to train at a particular hospital because they knew someone who was nursing there or because it was recommended to them by a friend, but only five men said they had a close relative nursing or working at the same hospital. We did not find any evidence to support the popular belief that recruitment of overseas nurses to particular hospitals is mostly a family affair.

SUMMARY

It seems odd to use the expression 'tradition-directed' in connection with such a non-traditional field for men as nursing; but it does look as if a proportion of the entrants were considerably influenced by the example of parents and relatives already in nursing. This would be consistent with what they said about the encouragement they had received from these sources. For the others (who are in the majority), the influence of friends seems to have been slight. They seem to have been 'inner-directed' in the sense that they reached an independent decision to look into the possibilities of nursing, some being attracted by extrinsic but most by intrinsic considerations. They did not receive (or perhaps seek) a great deal of help from official agencies. It is consistent with this interpretation that personal contacts played a smaller part (at least for the students) in the selection of a hospital than might be expected either from the other surveys quoted or from surveys about girls entering nursing. Many of them made contact with the training hospital through the impersonal device of a newspaper advertisement.

Career factors seemed to be less salient than we had expected for these entrants, except in the important but limited sense that they were looking forward to a significant improvement in their pay when they completed their training. Only 17% (dropping to 11% among general entrants and 6% among pupils) spontaneously mentioned promotion or career prospects as a reason for choosing to nurse. Almost as many mentioned security, which seemed to be what some of them meant by 'career'. But far more mentioned the satisfactions of nursing and the opportunity to help other people. Similarly only 11% (18% general, 8% mental illness, 4% mental subnormality) mentioned career factors among their reasons for choosing a particular field of nursing. And although the great majority said that the promotion prospects would encourage 'a man who was just wondering whether or not to take up nursing' (more so than any other aspect of nursing) only two-thirds of the students and less than half the pupils specifically said that they themselves had been encouraged by this factor.

To sum up this part of the discussion, it looks as if male entrants to nursing share with many of their contemporaries a desire for their work to be interesting and satisfying in itself, although they may feel the need for intrinsic job-satisfactions more strongly than others from comparable social and educational backgrounds. They are not unusual in giving relatively little weight to pay and security. They are, however, different from the majority of men of their age in expressing such a strong desire to help and work with people – attitudes normally found more often among women. Perhaps to some extent in conquence of this, some of them have had difficulty in settling down in a steady job in the past.

Recruitment, however, is a two-way process. The candidate has to choose the occupation, the field and a specific employer. The potential employer has to be prepared to accept the applicant. We therefore feel it right to conclude this chapter with a note about hospital attitudes to male recruitment as indicated to us in the interviews with senior staff.

Footnote on hospital attitudes to the recruitment of male nurses

Male students and pupils constituted nearly half the total trainees at mental illness and mental subnormality hospitals covered by the survey but only a small part of the intake to the general hospitals.

The psychiatric hospitals had virtually no restrictions on the recruitment of men, apart from the usual entrance requirements, although some reported having to accept men of a lower standard than they would wish because of shortages of suitable recruits in their area. Some said they discouraged married men from training and one MSN hospital liked its male recruits to be reasonably tall in order to be able to cope with aggressive patients. Otherwise it was only the general hospitals which imposed many restrictions on the recruitment of men. Two general hospitals claimed to have no restrictions, six said they were restricted only by the number of (male) beds and six by the limited availability of residential accommodation for men. However four hospitals said they looked for a higher standard in men than in women before taking them on and the other seven hospitals were obviously very wary about taking men at all. Several of the hospitals indicated that they considered male nurses to have only a limited role in general nursing and were not prepared to accept men for training who did not display at least as strong a motivation as their female recruits.

We were particularly interested in the attitudes of the hospitals which recruited male pupil nurses. There was a possibility that male pupils were mostly the rejects from student training. Three-quarters of those in our survey population had not applied to any other hospital for pupil training although over a quarter had been rejected for student training elsewhere. Many hospitals suggested to us that male pupils are often recruited just as 'pairs of hands' whatever their quality and qualifications. This situation may have been due not only to the hospital's staffing difficulties, but also to its quality as a training institution: we found that more pupils were recruited by hospitals in the lowest of the three categories assessed by the GNC inspectorate. But hospitals which employed their own entrance tests for student training also tended to recruit more male pupils. This suggested that, at least in some hospitals, male pupils were often student rejects. In other hospitals however it was clear that there was a real place for male pupils.

On overseas nurses, the information from hospitals showed that a variety of recruitment methods are employed. Many hospitals do not recruit direct from abroad, but others recruit from overseas without even an interview. Tutors often expressed scepticism as to the validity of some of their overseas recruits' qualifications, and some hospitals had imposed a ban on recruits from specific areas e.g. Mauritius. Others employed special tests of their own which they administered to overseas recruits. On the whole it seemed that the method of recruitment depended on the availability of local labour and on the tradition of a particular hospital. The Briggs Committee found serious fault with hospitals' approach to the recruitment of overseas nurses, and recommended a tightening up of selection arrangements and more adequate arrangements for their reception and induction.[17] We reached similar conclusions.[18]

REFERENCES
1. T. Veness, School Leavers, 1962.
2. Government Social Survey Young School Leavers: an Enquiry for the Schools Council, 1968.
3. P. H. Mann, Young Men and Work, University of Sheffield, Department of Sociological Studies, 1966.
4. M. Carter, Into Work, 1966.
5. R. V. Clements, The Choice of Careers by Schoolchildren, 1958.
6. D. C. Marsh and A. J. Willcocks, Focus on Nurse Recruitment, Nuffield Provincial Hospitals Trust, 1965.
7. Leeds Regional Hospital Board, unpublished report of a Survey of the attitudes of Girls aged 15–20, and others, towards nursing and hospitals in Huddersfield, 1965.
8. M. Scott-Wright, Student Nurses in Scotland: Characteristics of Success and Failure, Scottish Home and Health Department, 1968.
9. J. M. MacGuire, From Student to Nurse: Part I — The Induction Period, Oxford Area Nurse Training Committee, 1961.
10. Sheffield Regional Hospital Board, Nursing Cadet Schemes, (unpublished report), 1963.
11. Report of the Committee on Nursing (Cmnd. 5115, 1972) para. 191.
12. J. G. Rosen and K. Jones, 'The Male Nurse', New Society, 9th March, 1972, pp. 493–4.
13. Department of Health and Social Security (Statistics and Research Divison) Overseas born student and pupil nurses and pupil midwives in National Health Service Hospitals, at 31st December, 1968.
14. A. Singh, 'Why Nurses Nurse', Further Education, Vol. 2, No. 4 (Summer 1971) pp. 164–6.
15. Report of the Committee on Nursing, op. cit., para. 416.
16. ibid. para. 192.
17. ibid. paras. 323–6, 591, 714.
18. R. W. H. Stones 'Overseas Nurses in Britain: a study of male recruits', Nursing Times, Occasional Paper, 7th September, 1972, pp. 141–144.

5. IMAGES OF NURSING HELD BY MALE RECRUITS

In the two previous chapters we have examined the background characteristics of male entrants and the processes through which they came into nursing. We have also touched on the advantages and disadvantages of nursing, as they saw them, as a career for men. In this chapter we examine in more detail their image of their chosen profession and the shifts that occurred during their first year in training. The picture they gave us differed significantly both from attitudes and beliefs about nursing held by various groups in the general population and from the image held by female student nurses at a similar stage in their training. The chapter starts with a brief review of comparative material from earlier surveys.

PREVIOUS SURVEYS

General Population

In January 1968, a representative sample of over 2,000 adults was interviewed by National Opinion Polls on behalf of the Ministry of Health to obtain their opinions about nursing.[1] Although 'nursing' was not defined, most of the answers probably refer to *female* nurses.

Ninety-five per cent of those interviewed believed that nurses worked very hard, and three quarters believed that nurses worked harder than teachers, social workers or secretaries. Similarly large majorities believed that nurses worked longer hours and enjoyed shorter holidays than most other people.

Fifty-two per cent thought that nurses were underpaid and another 10% very underpaid. But 67% (ranging from 58% in the top AB class group to 75% in DE) agreed that 'nursing has very good career prospects'. (Some American work in the early 1950's suggested that the status and attractions of nursing are more highly regarded by lower socio-economic groups.)[2]

The majority believed that nursing was more worthwhile than any of a number of other suggested occupations (although a substantial minority of respondents under 35 voted for teaching) and that it was more respected in the community. Sixty-seven per cent would encourage – or strongly encourage – a teenage daughter to take up nursing if she wanted and 36% regarded nursing as the best job for a young girl to go into (more than e.g. teaching or secretarial work).

Eighty-nine per cent agreed that 'you have to have a vocation to be a nurse' and 75% agreed that 'nurses are competent self-possessed people' – much of the disagreement with both statements coming from those under 25. Eighty per cent did *not* agree that 'it is easy for any girl to become a nurse' and only 7% agreed that 'to take up nursing is a waste of a good education'. Nurses were thought (except by those under 25) to require more intelligence than civil servants, social workers, bank clerks and secretaries, but not so much as teachers or research workers.

The sample was about equally divided between those who agreed and disagreed with the statements 'nursing is an unpleasant job as you are always in contact with sick people' and 'hospitals are nice places to work in'. There was however an important age and sex difference here. Women and all respondents under 35 tended to disagree with the first statement whereas more men, more of the older people and more from classes DE agreed with it. Conversely, women tended to agree that hospitals were pleasant places to work in whereas men, and the younger respondents, disagreed.

Seventy-one per cent (76% of those under 35) agreed that 'nurses spend a lot of time doing chores'. Fifty per cent thought that 'nurses are subject to more discipline than necessary'. Only 25% agreed that 'nurses have a very attractive social life'.

Apart from their expressed dislike of hospitals as such, the male respondents, half the total, shared the same image of nursing as women. But (as in the American study already quoted) it was slightly more negative. Men were more inclined to say that nurses were under-paid and worked longer hours than average. Fewer thought that nursing was more respected and worthwhile than teaching. Slightly more thought that nursing was a waste of a good education and would discourage a teenage daughter from entering it. But these are minor differences of degree. The largest difference between men and women was in their attitude to career prospects: 32% of men (but only 20% women) disagreed with the statement that a nurse had very good career prospects.

Perhaps these answers would have been different if the respondents had been asked specifically about men in nursing. They would certainly have been different if they had been asked of men who were themselves considering a nursing career. Girls who take up nursing are entering a profession which is socially approved for them: a quarter of the general population think of nursing as a suitable first choice of career and about one girl in three contemplates taking up nursing at some time.[3] Nursing is a less obvious choice for men, and it would be surprising if their attitudes to the profession coincided with those of men in the general population.

Potential Female Recruits

Two local studies of girls in the potential recruitment range (ages 15 to 20) go more deeply than the previous survey and also make some attempt to see how the image held by girls who actually take up nursing differs from that of their contemporaries. One team, working in Mansfield in 1961–62, interviewed nearly 2,000 girls of whom about half were aged between 16 and 20 (including about 5% who were or had been nurses) and the rest were on the point of leaving school.[4] Another study, commissioned in 1966 by the Leeds Regional Hospital Board, covered 187 Huddersfield school leavers as well as 65 nurses who had recently left the service of local hospitals.[5] The Huddersfield study was deliberately based on the earlier one and used some of the same questions.

All groups held the popular image of nurses as overworked and underpaid. But more detailed questions showed that the non-nurses were not well informed about nursing conditions. They considerably under-estimated the pay that nurses actually enjoyed and seemed also to exaggerate the number of hours they worked: over half the Mansfield 16–20 year olds thought that a nurse worked over 46 hours a week, and a quarter thought it was more than 48 – the true figure at that time being 44.* They accorded high social standing to the nurses – below a lady doctor, slightly lower than a physiotherapist, slightly higher than a teacher or a worker in a children's home, considerably higher than shorthand typists, bank clerks, shop assistants, and themselves. They agreed that nurses had to be intelligent; and many had been put off nursing because they did not rate themselves intelligent enough for it.

The Mansfield girls were asked whether they saw nursing as a vocation, a career or a job. About two-thirds saw it as a career, supporting their choice by practical points like the opportunity to better oneself, long training, examinations and prospects. Only a fifth saw it as a vocation – explaining this with reference to the need for a nurse to like her job in spite of the conditions and unpleasantness – but this minority included most of the grammar school girls in the sample and about half the nurses. Very few, mostly from secondary modern schools, described it as a job.

* At the time of our survey nurses worked a standard 42 hours week; it was reduced to 40 at the end of 1972.

Both populations agreed with a number of complimentary statements about nurses (e.g. 'nurses are self-sacrificing') and disagreed with statements critical of internal hospital relationships (e.g. 'senior nurses are unpleasant to junior nurses' and 'hospital matrons are disliked by their nurses'). The nurses in the sample, however, were very critical of staff relationships and agreed with both the last two statements. Those who had relatives working in hospitals or who had been patients after the age of fifteen were also more critical than other girls. Interestingly enough, the ex-patients and those with relatives did not share the general view about nurses being over-worked; but they did accept a statement that 'Nurses often have to scrub floors' which the other girls overwhelmingly rejected. (Job-analyses carried out in 1950–53 show junior nurses spending about 5–10% of their time on work labelled 'domestic', i.e. not directly connected to the care of the patients; but this seems to have involved dusting and sweeping rather than scrubbing.)[6, 7]

There are then, differences between the perceptions of those who have some personal knowledge of nursing and those who have not. In the Huddersfield survey, respondents were asked to select from a list of 14 qualities the three they considered it most important for a nurse to have. The only qualities selected by more than half the non-nurses were 'calmness in emergencies' (mentioned by 57.2%) 'patience' (56.2%) and 'not likely to be upset by unpleasant sights, sounds or smells', (55.6%). (The other qualities, in declining order of importance, were 'love of other people', 'ability to accept discipline', 'intelligence', 'good temperament', 'practical skill', 'unselfishness', 'sense of humour', 'perseverance', 'energy', 'variety of interests' and 'high moral character'.) The list was much the same for ex-patients and for those whose parents had worked in hospital. Those whose mothers had worked as nurses did not differ much either, although they put more emphasis on practical skill and a sense of humour and put intelligence at the bottom of the list! But those who had themselves been nurses gave highest place, after patience (mentioned by 57.7%) to love of other people and ability to accept discipline (37.7% compared to 21.9% of the other teenagers, who put it in fifth place).

Female Student nurses – the Oxford Study

The most thorough analysis of the image of nursing held by students at the start of their training is in a longitudinal study of 292 girls who started student training at five general hospitals in the Oxford area in 1960–61.[8] Some of the recurring 'image' questions were first asked (at least in this country) in this study. For example, these students too were asked whether they would say nursing was a career or a vocation for them. Fifty-six per cent (compared with 45% of the nurses in the Mansfield study, some of whom were older while some had left nursing) said it was a vocation – which was taken to imply their acceptance that nursing involved a particular way of life – and 43% said it was a career.

They were also asked to describe the qualities of a good nurse and a bad nurse, and to say what they thought was the main aim of the nursing staff in a hospital. The author of the study was looking for evidence of identification with the profession and with the nursing ethic. She considered that a strongly identified girl would include technical nursing skills among the qualities of a good nurse. In fact only 38% thought that a good nurse had to be skilled and proficient at nursing procedures, and only 14% mentioned the lack of technical skill as an attribute of the bad nurse. Just under a third thought that a good nurse would be deeply interested in patients, but nearer half suggested that a bad nurse would not be. The majority distinguished between good and bad nurses in terms of personal qualities – sympathy, kindness and patience on the one hand, and laziness, unwillingness, ill humour on the other.

It was also suggested that those more identified with the profession would mention 'care' as the main aim of the nursing staff and be less likely to confuse nursing with medical 'curing' roles. About 60% gave the cure of patients as one of the main aims while just under half (with some overlap) mentioned the provision of care and comfort. A further pointer was thought to be whether the student nurse described herself mainly as a nurse or mainly as a student. The identified entrant would see herself mainly as a nurse. In fact, 86% of the girls saw themselves as students. There was therefore a difference between the way these students saw themselves and a 'professional' image of nursing.

Potential Schoolboy Recruits

The only indication we have of differences between boys' attitudes to nursing as a career for themselves and those of girls at the same age comes from a survey of pupils aged 15 to 16 in five suburban comprehensive schools in the Leicester area.[9] A questionnaire dealing with attitudes to nursing was given to a random sample of girls and to any boys who expressed interest when they were told about the enquiry. Although the 76 boys were self-selected only a minority of them were interested in nursing and only one seriously. The boys were in general more concerned with wages than girls, and less inclined to think that the career prospects in nursing were good.

Opinion Surveys for the Briggs Committee

The Committee on Nursing commissioned a number of research projects in 1970–71. A postal survey covered 5% of all hospital nursing and midwifery staff, including nursing auxiliaries, and 10% of corresponding staff in the community services. Eleven per cent of the hospital respondents were male and 22% were students or pupils. The postal inquiry was followed by 1655 personal interviews. Separate surveys were made of inactive nurses and midwives and of overseas nurses. The Committee found a high level of job-satisfaction but some dissatisfaction with the status of the individual nurse and, particularly among students and male nurses, with staff relations. The majority of students felt that they sometimes had to perform non-nursing 'chores' that more appropriately belong to messengers or domestic staff. Two-fifths of all hospital nurses and midwives agreed that doctors did not take enough account of nurses' skill and experience. Fifty-nine per cent of students complained of overwork and 61% of petty rules and discipline. Three-quarters of the students (two-thirds of the pupils) alleged that the level of responsibility varied too much from day to day. Nearly all the trainees agreed that 'senior nurses often forget what it was like to be a junior nurse'.[10]

MALE ENTRANTS TO NURSING – COMPARISON AND CONTRAST

A number of questions about image were incorporated in the questionnaires administered to male nurses. In interpreting the figures, it is necessary to keep in mind that whereas most of the other surveys deal with female student nurses in general hospitals, the male population included post-registration trainees and pupils as well as students, and entrants to the psychiatric fields as well as general. To avoid too many complicating factors, and to make the figures as comparable as possible with those of earlier surveys, the answers from post-registration students are shown separately in the tables and the main discussion is directed to the 466 students and pupils embarking on a basic training. (The effective total was reduced to 391 by the exclusion of Mauritian entrants from the analysis of certain questions, with which they clearly had difficulty in the first interview).

Nearly all the 'image' questions were asked twice – in the initial interview shortly after the start of training and again a year later. In the meantime, of course, some had left nursing and a small number of the others could not be re-interviewed for various reasons. Where appropriate, the tables show answers from both interviews, and include replies from experienced post-registration students in our sample (and, where relevant, from other surveys) for comparison. We have also noted any important differences between the replies at the first interview of those who did ('stayers') or did not ('leavers') complete the first year of training.

Self-image
In the NOP Survey[1] all but 20% of young people under 25 and all but 13% of men (all ages) had agreed that 'You need to have a vocation to be a nurse'.

Compared to female students and the Mansfield grammar school girls fewer of the men described nursing as a vocation but compared to the Mansfield secondary modern girls the men were more inclined to think nursing a vocation. Within our sample, as with the Mansfield girls, however, ex-grammar school boys were more likely to say nursing was a vocation (55%) than ex-secondary modern boys (37%). More entrants to general training said it was a vocation (45% against 39% in mental illness), but nursing was a job to more MSN entrants (14% against 6% in general and 8% in mental illness) and to more of the overseas students (18%). Those who entered training at 21 or over, those with previous hospital employment experience and those who confessed to doubts about the decision to nurse were all more likely to see nursing as a job (23% of those with serious doubts and 12.5% with slight doubts against 7% with no doubts). The same was true for those who left training in the first year (12.5% of leavers said it was a job compared with 7% of stayers).

Those entrants who said nursing was a career to them were more likely than the others to have included career or promotion prospects among their reasons for taking up nursing. They also put promotion prospects higher in importance in their decision to nurse. Fourteen per cent of those who said it was a job said they took up nursing because of being out of work or needing a job (compared with 5% who said vocation or career). Eleven per cent of the same group (against 4% who said vocation or career) gave 'poor career opportunities' as a reason why more men did not take up nursing.

Fewer of the pupils saw nursing as a career; but the difference between students and pupils was very small.

TABLE 5.1

Would you say that nursing is a vocation, a career or a job? (Asked at initial interview only)

	Voca- tion	Career	Job	Don't know	N = 100%
Students*	39%	50%	9%	2%	325
Pupils*	42%	45%	11%	2%	66
Post-registration students	21%	57%	21%	1%	76
Oxford – student nurses	56%	43%	—	1%	256
Mansfield – nurses	46%	50%	4%	—	24
– others					
,, aged 20	21%	64%	15%	—	284
,, aged 20 ex-grammar school	53%	40%	7%	—	53
,, aged 16–19 ex-grammar school	72%	25%	3%	—	152
,, aged 20 ex-sec. modern	15%	68%	17%	—	225
,, aged 16–19 ex-sec. modern	10%	80%	10%	—	274

* Excluding Mauritians.

More of the male entrants, but only a minority of students at the initial interview, identified as nurses. Those who described themselves as students were slightly more heavily represented among those who did not complete the first year (59% against 51%). Entrants to general training were more likely to see themselves as nurses (53%) while 62% of entrants to mental subnormality described themselves as students.

TABLE 5.2

How do you think of yourself at the moment?
- mainly as a *student* who is expected to do a great deal of practical work in the course of his training

or
- mainly as a *nurse* who is expected to do a great deal of theoretical study in the course of his work.

	Mainly as student	Mainly as nurse	Don't know	N = 100%
Students:				
– first interview*	55%	43%	2%	325
– second interview	39%	56%	5%	265
Pupils:				
– first interview*	44%	56%	—	66
– second interview	43%	57%	—	65
Post-registration students	56%	41%	3%	76
Oxford student nurses (before going on wards)	86%	12% †	2%	200

* Excluding Mauritians.
† This rose to 46% when the girls were interviewed again after they had started on ward work.

The majority of those who took part in the second interview (now including the Mauritians) described themselves, after a year in training, as nurses. The proportion who saw themselves mainly as students dropped in all fields to 37.5% in general, 43% in mental illness and 37% in MSN. (It should not generally be assumed that differences between the answers to the first and second interviews are due to individual shifts of opinion, since the populations are not the same and we are more concerned to show what a cross-section of nurses were thinking at a particular point in training. But in this case there does seem to have been some shift among students towards self-perception as 'mainly a nurse' during the year.)

TABLE 5.3

What, in your opinion, is the main aim of the nursing staff in a hospital; what are they there to do?

	% mentioning care of patient	% mentioning cure of patient	No.
Students:			
– first interview*	70%	42%	325
– second interview	75%	35%	265
Pupils:			
– first interview*	70%	36%	66
– second interview	75%	17%	65
Post-registration students	70%	51%	76
Oxford student nurses:			
(before going on wards)	46%	59%	200
(on ward)	50%	60%	200

* Excluding Mauritians.

The men in all fields were more likely to mention care than the Oxford girls. It was mentioned by 79% of the mental subnormality entrants, only 27% of whom mentioned cure. Cure was mentioned most by those in mental illness (48% compared to 38% in general). Overseas entrants were least likely to mention it.

After a year in training care came up in threequarters of the interviews. Fewer mentioned cure, particularly among the pupils. There was still a marked field difference. At the second interview only 18% of MSN entrants mentioned cure (against 36% in general and mental illness) and 88% mentioned care (against 73% in general and 70% in mental illness).

Professional development

TABLE 5.4

In your first year how much do you think your work on the wards will differ from the work of a Registered Staff Nurse.* Will it differ in skill or responsibility or both? (* State Enrolled Nurse for pupil respondents.)

	No differ-ence or don't know	Differ in skill	Differ in responsi-bility	Differ in both	N = 100%
Students:					
– first interview	4%	7%	11%	78%	372
– second interview	5%	8%	22%	65%	265
Pupils:					
– first interview	14%	8%	16%	62%	94
– second interview	32%	6%	18%	44%	65
Post-registration nurses	3%	9%	26%	62%	76
Oxford student nurses†					
(before going on wards)	23%	47%	17%	13%	200
(on wards)	9%	69%	7%	15%	200

†The actual question asked was: 'How do you think your work on the wards will differ from what is done by the senior nurses?'

Perhaps this question was badly worded, and invited the respondents to go for both answers. It is therefore interesting that rather more of those who did choose opted for 'responsibility' (as did the post-registration students) whereas the Oxford girls were more inclined to mention 'skill' – overwhelmingly so once they were on the wards.

At the second interview an even greater percentage opted for 'responsibility'. But pupils were more inclined to say there was no difference. More general entrants saw no difference (16% as against 9% in mental illness and 7% in MSN). Slightly more of the entrants to the psychiatric fields saw the difference in terms of skill (10% as against 5% in general).

How would you describe a good nurse?

In answer to this question, 89% of the Oxford girls had mentioned 'personal' qualities, 31% interest in the patient and 38% nursing skills. The majority of the men, too, described a good nurse in terms of personal qualities (e.g. 'humane', 'sympathetic', 'patient with people') and about a third mentioned conscientiousness and dedication. Practical skill was specifically mentioned by only 5%, but over a quarter stipulated that a nurse should be efficient or knowledgeable.

The men were then shown a list of eight personal qualities and asked which one was (a) the most important (b) the next important and (c) the least important for a nurse to have. Their order of preference was quite clear: –

TABLE 5.5

Qualities of a good nurse?

	% regarding as most important*		% regarding as least important	
	First interview N = 391†	Second interview N = 330	First interview N = 391†	Second interview N = 330
Patient with people	34%	34%	1%	1%
Calm in emergencies	16%	21%	4%	4%
Practical skill	12%	7%	7%	8%
Intelligent	10%	13%	10%	8%
Shows initiative	10%	10%	6%	10%
Unselfish	9%	7%	19%	18%
Works hard	4%	4%	10%	15%
Able to accept discipline	3%	3%	36%	33%
Don't know	1%	—	5%	3%

* The preference rankings were not altered by including second choices.
† Excluding Mauritians.

There were differences between entrants to different fields: 'practical skill' was first or second choice for 36% of general entrants, 25% of MSN but only 23% of mental illness entrants. 'Patience with people' was chosen first or second by 59% in mental illness, 56% in MSN but only 38% in general. A tenth of the general entrants gave first choice to 'works hard', as against 3% of mental illness and MSN entrants. One in eight of the general entrants thought 'initiative' was the most important; but as many rated it least important. But all those groups agreed that the two least important qualities were 'unselfishness' and the 'ability to accept discipline'. There were no changes of any substance at the second interview.

In the Huddersfield survey, former nurses and school leavers had been asked to choose the top three most important qualities from a list of fourteen. All groups put patience and calmness near the top of the list. The ex-nurses in Huddersfield put a stronger emphasis on the ability to accept discipline. Rigid discipline, however, found few supporters among the students and pupils interviewed for the Briggs Committee.

Following this broad question, the men were asked whether they agreed or disagreed with a number of statements about nursing, some of which specifically concerned the qualities of the nurse and the possibility that they could be taught.

TABLE 5.6

A nurse needs to be very intelligent

	Agree	Disagree	Can't say	N = 100%
Students:				
– first interview	35%	62%	3%	372
– second interview	34%	63%	3%	265
Pupils:				
– first interview	55%	42%	3%	94
– second interview	54%	44%	2%	65
Post-registration students	37%	56%	7%	76
Nurses are very intelligent				
20 yr. old Mansfield girls	71%	22%	7%	312
Nurses are intelligent				
16–19 yr. old Mansfield girls	89%	6%	5%	1,094
Most nurses are very clever				
Huddersfield school leavers	51%	45%	4%	187

The men did not share the general belief (echoed in the NOP surveys of the general population) that intelligence is an important quality for a nurse. Rather more of the pupils, however, agreed with the statement. It has to be borne in mind that some of them may have been rejected for student nurse training on intellectual grounds. The British entrants, especially the younger ones, were more inclined to disagree with the statement than those from overseas.

TABLE 5.7

Nurses are very self-sacrificing

	Agree	Disagree	Can't say	N = 100%
Students:				
– first interview	47%	47%	6%	372
– second interview	45%	52%	3%	265
Pupils:				
– first interview	72%	22%	6%	94
– second interview	70%	25%	5%	65
Post registration students	43%	53%	4%	76
Nurses are self-sacrificing				
20 yr. old Mansfield girls	66%	24%	10%	317
Huddersfield school leavers	73%	17%	10%	187

More pupils than students agreed that nurses were very self-sacrificing. Entrants to mental illness differed from the other two in that only 45% agreed with the statement against 59% of general entrants and 60% of MSN. Most of the overseas entrants agreed with it. Among British entrants, it was accepted by rather more (but still a minority) of those who had themselves been hospital patients. There was slightly more disagreement at the second interview, and among post-registration students. But the initial differences persisted between students and pupils, and between British and overseas entrants.

TABLE 5.8

Nurses are born not made

	Agree	Disagree	Can't say	N = 100%
Students:				
– first interview	22%	74%	4%	372
– second interview	20%	75%	5%	265
Pupils:				
– first interview	48%	45%	7%	94
– second interview	37%	57%	6%	65
Post-registration students	22%	75%	3%	76
20 yr.-old Mansfield girls	46%	40%	14%	317
Huddersfield school leavers	46%	43%	11%	187

Although most of the men (particularly those in student training) rejected this statement, with its implication that nursing was not a communicable skill, a substantial minority agreed with it even at the second interview and post-registration stages. More overseas than British entrants agreed with it. (The Briggs Committee commented that this was 'perhaps the most stillborn of all the stereotypes')[11].

TABLE 5.9

Nursing runs in families

	Agree	Disagree	Can't say	N = 100%
Students:				
– first interview	24%	70%	6%	372
– second interview	37%	60%	3%	265
Pupils:				
– first interview	34%	63%	3%	94
– second interview	38%	60%	2%	65
Post-registration students	30%	65%	5%	76
20 yr.-old Mansfield girls	31%	59%	10%	317

The same pattern applied here. Again, more overseas entrants agreed that nursing ran in families. Those who had close family connections with nursing were more likely to agree than the others. There was a marked increase from 30% to 48% between first and second interviews in the proportion of MSN entrants who agreed with the statement. Since there were fewer nurses with family connections in the second interview population the increase in the percentage agreeing with the statement is rather surprising.

The Working Environment
Some of the other statements which were offered in this question

concerned the work of nurses and internal staff relationships in hospitals.

TABLE 5.10

Nurses are very overworked

	Agree	Disagree	Can't say	N = 100%
Students:				
– first interview	48%	44%	8%	372
– second interview	61%	35%	4%	265
Pupils:				
– first interview	54%	42%	4%	94
– second interview	77%	18%	5%	65
Post-registration students	72%	24%	4%	76
Nurses seem to be very overworked				
– Mansfield 16–19 girls	77%	16%	7%	1,091
Nurses are overworked				
– Huddersfield school leavers	69%	20%	11%	187

At the initial interview, less than half the students agreed with the popular belief about overwork. (It will be recalled, moreover, that the Mansfield girls with actual hospital contact or experience were less inclined to agree with this statement). The statement was rejected by relatively more British entrants, especially older men and those who had worked in a hospital before starting their training. The greater measure of agreement at the later interview, and among post-registration students, is therefore paradoxical and hard to explain. The nurses' pay campaign, which emphasized overwork and under-remuneration, reached an unprecedented level of militancy during 1969 and may have stimulated discontent among these men.

In general, pupils took a more 'idealistic' view of nurses (i.e., self-sacrificing and hard-working) than the students.

TABLE 5.11

Nurses often have to clean floors

	Agree	Disagree	Can't say	N = 100%
Students:				
– first interview	50%	43%	7%	372
– second interview	56%	42%	2%	265
Pupils:				
– first interview	60%	37%	3%	94
– second interview	55%	43%	2%	65
Post-registration students	52%	46%	2%	76
Nurses often have to scrub floors				
Mansfield 16–19 year old girls	30%	64%	6%	1,088
Huddersfield school leavers	27%	63%	10%	187
Nurses spend a lot of time doing chores				
Men (all ages)	71%	17%	12%	1,019
Young people 16–24 (both sexes)	76%	15%	9%	376

We were unable to adopt the form of this question used in earlier surveys. Pilot interviews showed that the word 'scrub' was too strong and would have led to the statement being overwhelmingly rejected by male students and pupils. The change in wording may have affected the replies: job analysis shows that nurses do in fact have domestic duties. (Again, it is worth remembering that the Mansfield girls who had been nurses or patients were more inclined than the others to accept the statement, even in its stronger version.) Within our sample, it was accepted by more of those who had previously worked in a hospital and by more psychiatric than general entrants – a difference which persisted in the second interview.

TABLE 5.12

Junior nurses spend a lot of time running errands

	Agree	Disagree	Can't say	N = 100%
Students:				
– first interview	53%	38%	9%	372
– second interview	60%	38%	2%	265
Pupils:				
– first interview	39%	53%	8%	94
– second interview	60%	40%	—	65
Post-registration students	66%	28%	6%	76

Again, the statement was accepted by more of those with hospital experience. It was accepted by 59% of MSN entrants at the first interview but only about half in the mental illness field and 41% in general. There was more agreement from general entrants by the second interview.

TABLE 5.13

Junior nurses are treated like children by the senior nurses

	Agree	Disagree	Can't say	N = 100%
Students:				
– first interview	36%	58%	6%	372
– second interview	42%	55%	3%	265
Pupils:				
– first interview	34%	59%	7%	94
– second interview	58%	40%	2%	65
Post-registration students	72%	21%	7%	76
Nurses are treated like children by their seniors				
Huddersfield school leavers	30%	55%	15%	187
Senior nurses are unpleasant to junior nurses				
Mansfield 16–19 year old girls	25%	62%	13%	1,083

This and the following questions were concerned with authority relationships and discipline. On nearly all of them, the second interview discovered more *unfavourable* attitudes than the first. The frequency of unfavourable answers from post-registration students is also noteworthy. (In the Mansfield survey, unfavourable statements of this sort were more likely to be accepted by former nurses and ex-patients).

TABLE 5.14

There are a lot of petty restrictions in hospitals

	Agree	Disagree	Can't say	N = 100%
Students:				
– first interview	59%	36%	5%	372
– second interview	77%	21%	2%	265
Pupils:				
– first interview	54%	40%	6%	94
– second interview	78%	20%	2%	65
Post-registration students	85%	13%	2%	76

Nurses are subject to more discipline than necessary				
Men (all ages)	49%	40%	11%	1,019
Young people aged 16–24 (both sexes)	51%	39%	10%	376

Only 61% of the students and nurses in the Briggs investigations agreed that 'nursing is hindered by petty rules and discipline': male respondents in that survey were generally more critical than female.

In answer to another question 43% of the students (excluding the Mauritians) said that they thought hospital discipline would discourage a man who was thinking of taking up nursing (36% gave neutral replies and 21% said it would encourage a potential entrant). However, only a third of the same students said that hospital discipline had influenced their own decision and half of these were actually encouraged by it; it is not clear whether this was because the respondents liked discipline or because there was not much of it, e.g. in psychiatric hospitals.

More of those with hospital employment experience agreed with the statement about petty restrictions at the initial interview. On the other hand, so did more of those under 21. In the case of younger entrants, agreement probably reflected a general dislike of restrictions, while for the older more experienced entrants it probably reflected their greater knowledge of what went on in hospitals.

TABLE 5.15

Doctors do not respect nurses

	Agree	Disagree	Can't say	N = 100%
Students:				
– first interview	21%	65%	14%	372
– second interview	28%	65%	7%	265
Pupils:				
– first interview	10%	83%	7%	94
– second interview	29%	62%	9%	65
Post-registration students	28%	61%	11%	76
Mansfield 16–19 year old girls	12%	81%	7%	1,065

74

The majority of male entrants thought that doctors did respect nurses, although rather more unfavourable views were expressed at the second interview. The statement was rejected by more of the men who had hospital employment experience (whereas in the Mansfield study those with recent experience as patients were more inclined to accept it). Pupils and overseas entrants were more inclined to take the idealistic view in the first interview.

The apparently small change between the two interviews conceals a remarkable switch of position between fields. From being *least* likely to agree with the statement at the first interview the general entrants became *most* likely to agree with it by the second. The percentage agreeing went up from 12 % to 33%, whereas the percentage of mental illness entrants who agreed rose only from 19% to 29% and the percentage in mental subnormality actually went down from 25% to 19%.

Attitudes to authority

TABLE 5.16

A good chief male nurse is unpopular	Agree	Disagree	Can't say	N = 100%
Students:				
– first interview	22%	70%	8%	372
– second interview	21%	76%	3%	265
Pupils:				
– first interview	24%	70%	6%	94
– second interview	22%	75%	3%	65
Post-registration students	26%	72%	2%	76
Chief male nurses are disliked by their nurses				
Students:				
– first interview	13%	71%	16%	372
– second interview	20%	74%	6%	265
Pupils:				
– first interview	11%	82%	7%	94
– second interview	17%	78%	5%	65
Post-registration students	16%	75%	9%	76
Hospital matrons are disliked by their nurses				
Students:				
– first interview	37%	45%	18%	372
– second interview	42%	45%	13%	265
Pupils:				
– first interview	11%	81%	8%	94
– second interview	24%	68%	8%	65
Post-registration students	39%	52%	9%	76
(Mansfield 16–19 year old girls	27%	58%	15%	1,067)
It is difficult for a man to work under a woman				
Students:				
– first interview	56%	39%	5%	372
– second interview	40%	48%	12%	265
Pupils:				
– first interview	42%	52%	6%	94
– second interview	34%	58%	8%	65
Post-registration students	67%	29%	4%	76

Table 5.16 covers a complex set of questions (not asked in that order) designed to try and distinguish a general feeling about hospital discipline from specific attitudes to female superiors (which might not, of course, be a problem in psychiatric hospitals with separate male and female wings). The different reaction to identical statements about the unpopularity of matrons and chief male nurses is interesting, particularly as the statement about male chiefs was often accepted reluctantly and the one about matrons agreed to with emphasis! The different situations in different fields of nursing may be important: only 16% of general entrants agreed that hospital matrons were disliked by their nurses (73% disagreed and 9% did not know) whereas entrants to other fields were more evenly divided. Similarly 60% of general entrants disagreed with the statement that it was difficult for a man to work under a woman, which was agreed to by 61% in mental illness and 56% in MSN. (In answer to another question the students were evenly divided among those who thought that 'the fact that most nurses are women' would encourage potential entrants, discourage them or have no influence. However only a quarter had been influenced themselves by the fact, just over half of these having been encouraged by it).

At the second interview, entrants to the psychiatric fields were more likely to agree that chief male nurses are disliked and general entrants to agree that matrons are disliked by their nurses. To some extent this is because many had been unable to offer any opinion at the first interview. But there is also a movement away from an idealistic position, at least among the pupils, who did not initially differentiate between matrons and chief male nurses as the students did.

Overseas students were least likely to accept any of the unfavourable statements about superiors. Among British entrants, those with employment or family contacts were most disposed to *reject* all three statements about the unpopularity of chief nursing officers. But a remarkable proportion of post-registration students agreed with the statements.

Pay

TABLE 5.17

Nurses are very underpaid	Agree	Disagree	Can't say	N = 100%
Students:				
− first interview	75%	21%	4%	372
− second interview	88%	10%	2%	265
Pupils:				
− first interview	67%	26%	7%	94
− second interview	89%	9%	2%	65
Post-registration students	84%	12%	4%	76

Do you think nurses in general are very well paid, well paid, average, underpaid or very underpaid?

	Very well paid	Well paid	Aver- age	Under- paid	Very under- paid	Don't know	N = 100%
Men (all ages)	—	2%	25%	56%	12%	5%	2,135
Young people 16–24 (both sexes)	—	2%	34%	49%	9%	6%	376

Two-fifths of the hospital nurses and midwives in the Briggs survey gave first or second place to 'more basic pay' among their priorities for improvement in working conditions.

Whereas many of the general public express the view that nurses are underpaid without having any accurate picture of the scales of pay currently in force, the men in our sample were of course perfectly aware of what a nurses's pay was. Younger entrants were as likely as their elders to agree that nurses were underpaid.

Overseas entrants were more likely than the British to disagree at the first interview, but many changed their minds during the year. This may reflect changes in their reference groups.

The proportion who agreed with the statement had risen significantly by the second interviews in 1969, and at that stage included relatively more psychiatric than general entrants, in spite of the fact that psychiatric nurses enjoyed a salary 'lead'.

Social status

We have noted the high estimation of a nurse's social standing by the general population in comparison with teaching, social work and similar occupations. American nurses also estimate their own status high in comparison with these other occupations. We wanted to know how the male entrants ranked themselves, and also whether they gave the same social status to male and female nurses. To avoid cultural complications affecting people from overseas, this part of the analysis refers only to British entrants.

In reply to a general question 67% of these entrants had said the social standing of a nurse would encourage a potential applicant. (Only 15% said it would discourage him – and 40% said it encouraged *them*).

The entrants were asked to estimate how a qualified male nurse (*sc.* an enrolled nurse in the case of pupils) compared for social standing with a number of other specified occupations, three of which are classed by the Registrar-General in Social Class II (the same as a qualified nurse) and five in Class III. Here are the results. (The occupations are not in the order in which they were asked).

In general, the students put the qualified male nurse into the same social class as the Registrar-General did, but not so high as the ratings given to nurses by the general population. They put the qualified nurse well below probation officers, somewhat lower than physio-therapists, and about the same level as school teachers (whose esti-mated status seems to drop as respondents themselves drop in the social scale), somewhat higher than bank clerks and army sergeants and considerably higher than factory foremen and skilled manual operatives.

TABLE 5.18

Social status of male nurses

Compared with:	British students (273) Registered male nurse is:			British pupils (50) Male enrolled nurse is:		
	Lower	About same	Higher	Lower	About same	Higher
(Class II)						
Probation officer	53%	43%	4%	58%	34%	8%
Physiotherapist	45%	42%	13%	56%	26%	18%
School teacher	30%	63%	7%	52%	42%	6%
(Class III)						
Bank clerk	20%	43%	37%	26%	28%	46%
Army sergeant	13%	36%	51%	24%	38%	38%
Factory foreman	12%	29%	59%	22%	36%	42%
Fitter	3%	18%	79%	4%	34%	62%
Garage mechanic (Class IV if unskilled)	2%	20%	78%	—	32%	68%

Pupils were more modest about the status of the qualified enrolled nurse but their answers follow the same general pattern.

The men were also asked how they thought a qualified *female* nurse compared for social standing with some other female occupa-tions. For obvious reasons the two lists could not be exactly comparable but the results, which are given below, indicate that men give about the same status to female nurses as to male nurses when comparing them to physiotherapists and probation officers, and put female nurses slightly higher when comparing them to school teachers and bank clerks.

TABLE 5.19

Social status of female nurses

	British students (273) Qualified female nurse is:			British pupils (50) Enrolled female nurse is:		
	Lower	About same	Higher	Lower	About same	Higher
(Class II)						
Probation officer	54%	42%	4%	56%	34%	10%
Physiotherapist	45%	44%	11%	46%	34%	20%
School teacher	27%	65%	8%	40%	50%	10%
(Class III)						
Private secretary	22%	32%	46%	30%	26%	44%
Bank clerk	12%	42%	46%	32%	24%	44%
Hairdresser	3%	14%	83%	6%	18%	76%
(Class IV)						
Shop assistant	—	6%	94%	6%	12%	82%

In answer to identical questions, the students taking part in the second interview gave the same relative positions, except that physiotherapists now came slightly below teachers; but the comparative rankings were slightly less favourable to the registered male nurse. Only 31 British pupils were still training at that time and the number is too small for useful comparison with the results of the first interview.

The post-registration students gave a qualified male nurse lower status overall. As well as the three occupations rated higher by the pre-registration students they gave bank clerks higher social standing than a nurse (and indeed higher than physiotherapists). School teachers came second in their ratings, i.e. even higher than for the pre-registration students and very much higher than for the Mansfield girls, who put a teacher below a qualified female nurse.

DISCUSSION

Many of the American studies of nursing have concentrated on two apparently conflicting images. 'At one pole is the image of the humanitarian and altruistic person, more or less competent and endowed with sympathy, compassion, and exceptional capacities for establishing rapport – one who gives of herself. At the other pole is the image of the professional, well-trained, technically efficient, and coolheaded individual who can be relied upon for able performance within her specialty, and relatively independent of feeling components – one who may seem to keep herself out of her work'.[12] One American report found that as nurses progressed through their training they started by seeing the ideal nurse in personal, non-technical terms and only gradually began to judge her by technical and professional criteria.

It would be fair to sum up the British public's image as one heavily weighted towards personal qualities – intelligence, hard work and self-sacrifice – although nursing is also seen, particularly by women and by lower socio-economic groups, as offering good career prospects. Research among potential recruits suggests that this picture of the nurse can easily become idealized to an extent that may discourage suitable candidates. Those who do enter the profession seem to see themselves primarily in a helping role. Dr MacGuire's studies in Oxford found little evidence of a shift to less personal, more professional criteria of self-assessment during training.

It is convenient to approach our own data in terms of the *a priori* assumptions behind our questionnaire. We expected to find that the men who actually entered nursing would differ both from the general population and from female entrants in the following respects:

(a) they would see nursing more in terms of a career and less as a vocation;

(b) they would be more inclined to describe nursing in terms of technical than of personality requirements;
(c) they would be less likely to hold an idealized image of a nurse;
(d) their attitude to discipline would be less hierarchical (i.e. they would be less tolerant of unnecessary rules but more sympathetic to the problems of higher-level staff);
(e) they would expect to have problems with superiors of the opposite sex.

These expectations were partially, but not entirely, fulfilled. The picture was complicated by differences between entrants to different fields of nursing, and by differences between British students on the one hand and overseas entrants and pupils on the other.

Nursing as a career

Although a substantial minority described nursing as a vocation, far more men described it as a career or a job. It is uncertain how far this and other differences from female entrants were due to sheer maleness and how far to the greater age and maturity of the male entrants. Another factor might have been social class: their approach to some aspects of nursing was linked to school background, those from grammar schools being more likely in this case to talk of a vocation.

The general picture that emerged was of a career which offered poor financial rewards but adequate status and promotion prospects. One did not have to be born or called to be a nurse! But other questions suggested that the main appeal of nursing lay in the intrinsic nature of the work and it could be that men needed the career image to rationalize and legitimize (to themselves and their peers) their decision to enter a field that, as they themselves said, was not thought of as a man's job and was moreover poorly paid. It is significant that more who described it as a job failed to last the first year. On the other hand fully a fifth of the post-registration students (who tended to hold a less favourable image of their profession than the new entrants) also described nursing as a job.

Nursing as a technical skill

It has been suggested that male nurses fit particularly well into a technical rather than a comfort role.[13] But our male entrants were even more inclined than the Oxford girls to describe a good nurse in terms of personal qualities rather than as the possessor of communicable skills. Nor did they put practical skill high among the essential qualities of a nurse. Idealistic qualities like self-sacrifice and industry did not come very high either; patience and calmness, which came top of the list, suggested professional detachment and competence rather than moral virtue. There is also a professional feel about their emphasis on the greater responsibility as well as skill of the qualified nurse. Post-registration students were the most likely to describe the difference between their own work and that of a qualified nurse in terms of responsibility (whereas many pupils doubted whether there was any difference between their duties and those of a qualified enrolled nurse).

So the general picture here is one of a competent, responsible person rather than of one skilled in technical procedures. There is no need for a nurse to be a saint; but a seasoning of the saintly virtues, or their absence, affects the ability of a nurse to perform in that role.

The realism of the image

Our reasoning here was that men would have gone more carefully than girls into the true situation before starting training. If their image was excessively idealistic or unrealistic, however, we would be able to detect a change of view as a result of experience. There ought therefore to be something like a continuum of realism, with experienced post-registration nurses at the most realistic end, completely inexperienced new entrants at the other, and in the middle those with previous family or employment contacts and those who were interviewed after a year in training. And so it turned out, except of course that the post-registration image tended to be a 'mental illness' one, since most of the post-registration students had originally trained in that field.

One of the exceptions was the question about whether the respondent saw himself mainly as a student or as a nurse. Although far more men than women entrants described themselves as nurses at the first interview, and there was a further movement in that direction by the second interview, the post-registration students were just as likely as the pre-registration starters to identify themselves as students. Perhaps in this case their answers were influenced by the transition to a more learning role after holding qualified nurse status.

There was a definite progression in the answers to most of the questions about a nurse's duties and the qualities needed to perform them. The more experienced the respondent, the less likely he was to claim that nurses were very self-sacrificing and the more likely he was to agree that junior nurses were treated like children by senior nurses and that hospitals were full of petty restrictions. In all these respects, the men started with a less idealistic view than the general population.

They were more realistic than female entrants in appreciating the caring role of the nurse. Even the general entrants, who were more like their female counterparts in many ways, mentioned cure far less often than the Oxford girls. This feeling of realism came out even in the differences between fields. The mental subnormality entrants placed a particularly strong emphasis on care (and indeed on self-sacrifice) while curative functions were mentioned most frequently by those in mental illness training where surely the nurse has the most therapeutic role. It also seemed realistic that those in both the psychiatric fields

F

should emphasize the nurse's need for patience, whereas general entrants were more likely to mention practical skills.

We conclude, therefore, (a) that many of the critical statements about staff relationships and about nurses' duties were true and (b) that the male entrants in our sample had a more realistic picture of this sort of thing, even at the start of their training, than the general population. The main exception to this was the question about overwork. Nurses started with a more *favourable* picture than the general public but changed their views later in their careers. They may have been stimulated by the emphasis on overwork in the 'raise the roof' campaign to secure a pay increase, which was in progress at the time of the interviews.

The pupils, and the entrants from overseas, started with a more conventional image (e.g. of doctor/nurse relationships) than the others. They were more inclined to say that nurses needed high intelligence and moral qualities, and were less ready to agree with statements critical of internal staff relationships. It is a disquieting possibility that their greater reverence for the concept of a nurse stemmed from feelings of inferiority and inability to identify fully with nurses from their role as pupils. Many of them had already decided to take the full training for registration later on.

Attitudes to superiors

The assumption that men would have a more confident approach to senior staff of their own sex was based on nothing more than a hunch that women are more accultured to be submissive. In the event, we could not test our assumption owing to the dearth of comparative material about British female nurses. The evidence from our own survey is that men (especially post-registration nurses) are impatient of minor manifestations of authority and grow more so as their training proceeds. They do not think it is important for a nurse to be able to accept discipline. On the other hand they do not on the whole agree that chief male nurses either are or ought to be unpopular. Their feelings about *female* superiors are rather different.

Attitudes to women

We expected that even after they had taken the decision to enter what is still primarily a female world, except in the separately administered wings of psychiatric hospitals, male entrants would find it difficult to accept the reversal of the normal sex-roles by working under female superiors. In earlier hospital studies, Scott-Wright[14] and Woodward[15] noted that male nurses tended to become a rather defensive minority group and we thought that any such tendency would be emphasized by the small numbers of male entrants at the general hospitals in our sample.

The students did differentiate sharply between male and female chiefs, many holding with some vehemence that the latter (but not the former) were unpopular with their nurses and that it was difficult for a man to work under a woman. This view was not, however, shared by so many of the general entrants, who were most likely to meet female superiors early in their career. A year's experience somewhat softened the objections to female superiors but there was more criticism of both male and female chiefs in the second interview, although the difference between them remained. Pupils and overseas entrants, who tended to make light of relationships between the sexes in the first interview, were as likely as the others to agree with critical statements at the second.

We note also the degree of hostility to women shown by the post-registration nurses (some of whom were perhaps meeting them as competitors for the first time after transferring from psychiatric to general nursing) and the tendency to ascribe a slightly higher social status to female than to male nurses. Both these results suggest a feeling that men were at a disadvantage.

SUMMARY

Compared with female nurses and with the general population, therefore, these male entrants had a more down to earth image of nursing. They were bothered about pay and status, particularly in relation to female nurses, and were more likely to think in career than in vocational terms. They started training with a more realistic picture of what hospital life is like and did not share the popular view of the nurse as a paragon of virtue, self-sacrifice and unremitting industry. On the other hand, their image of the ideal nurse was rather like a male Florence Nightingale, dealing with patients in a sympathetic, competent, and responsible way. Although less personally involved in their work than female nurses, the men were far from seeing themselves as impersonal nursing technicians.

There are two practical implications in our findings which are important both for recruitment and for the training of male nurses.

(a) The image of nursing held by the general population is not likely to encourage a man to enter the profession who has a realistic picture of his own needs, strengths and failings. It is too idealized and perhaps too feminized. Hence the high proportion of male recruits who have derived a different image from family contacts and perhaps, too, the substantial minority who hold that nursing runs in families. If the public image was more like that held by the men in our sample, it would help to reassure those who would enjoy nursing but do not like the idea of working in a world dominated by female values.

(b) The implication for training is that it may not be possible to treat male and female students as completely interchangeable. Even in general hospitals the men take a somewhat different view from women about their profession and the demands it will make on them.

This image is in some ways more empirical and practical (e.g. their greater readiness to identify with a nursing role). The difference does not affect their suitability for training and if anything enhances their potential as trained nurses.

REFERENCES

1. National Opinion Polls Limited, *Attitudes to Nursing*, 1968 (unpublished report made available by the Department of Health and Social Security).
2. Summarized in L. W. Simmons and V. Henderson, *Nursing Research: a survey and reassessment*, 1964.
3. J. M. MacGuire, *Threshold to Nursing*, 1969.
4. D. C. Marsh and A. J. Willcocks, *Focus on Nurse Recruitment*, Nuffield Provincial Hospitals Trust 1965.
5. Leeds Regional Hospital Board, unpublished report of a *Survey of the Attitudes of girls aged 15–20, and others, towards nursing and hospitals in Huddersfield*, 1965.
6. Nuffield Provincial Hospitals Trust, *The Work of Nurses in Hospital Wards: Report of a Job-Analysis*, 1953.
7. Manchester Regional Hospital Board, *The Work of the Mental Nurse*, 1955.
8. J. M. MacGuire, *From Student to Nurse Part I — The Induction Period* Oxford Area Nurse Training Committee, 1961; *Part II — Training and Qualification*, 1966.
9. D. F. Clark, *A Survey of Attitudes to nursing among comprehensive School pupils in Leicestershire*, (duplicated report for Leicester No. 4 Hospital Management Committee, 1967).
10. Report of the Committee on Nursing (Cmnd. 5115) 1972, paras. 65–70, 107–110, 147, 229–30 and Appendix I.
11. *ibid.*, para. 103.
12. Simmons and Henderson, *op. cit.*, p. 222.
13. M. Olivie, 'The Male Nurse and Nursing', *Ons Ziekenhuis* (Holland), Vol. 27, No. 6 (June, 1965) pp. 181–190.
14. M. Scott-Wright, *Student Nurses in Scotland: Characteristics of Success and Failure*, Scottish Home and Health Department, 1968, p. 114.
15. J. Woodward, *Employment Relations in a Group of Hospitals*, 1960, p. 70.

In the previous chapters we looked at the means through which the men were recruited into nursing and the attitudes and images which they brought with them. We now examine the way they reacted, one year later, to their experience as trainees and how at that time they viewed the place of men in nursing. In the middle section of the chapter we look at the reasons why some men withdrew from training. (Altogether 210 entrants, 39% of the total, failed to complete their training, 60% of these withdrawing in the first year).

REACTIONS TO TRAINING[1]

General Reactions

Most of the men started nursing with the desire to help other people. Extrinsic rewards had not weighed heavily in their decision to nurse, although the opportunity to acquire new knowledge and skills was important to some. We expected that they would find most satisfaction in those aspects of their experience which involved close contact with patients and gave some meaning to their work.

The majority did in fact say that they had enjoyed their first year's training and derived satisfaction from meeting and helping people. The educational aspects of training were most appreciated by those without educational qualifications. The mental illness trainees expressed particular satisfaction with the opportunities for close patient contact.

Hardly any of the men specifically told us that they had liked the conditions of work but there was evidence to suggest that they found some aspects of these agreeable. Night duty for instance was preferred by a number of the men, notably because of the extra responsibility it gave them. However certain features were the cause of much dissatisfaction and led to preoccupation with extrinsic aspects of nursing. Pay was the major one of these, along with the irregularity of hours and particularly split shifts. There was some dissatisfaction, particularly in MSN hospitals, with overwork and having to do domestic and routine jobs. Most of these dissatisfactions have cropped up in studies of female recruits. The main difference between those and our findings was the men's concern with pay and their relative inability to manage on their training allowances.

More important than conditions of work was the relationship between members of staff in the hospitals. More men, especially in general hospitals, complained about these and the consequent lack of communication than about anything else. Also many were concerned about their own status and felt that senior nurses did not treat trainees with enough respect.

Problems of Adjustment

Like the girls in the Oxford study[2] the men had been most worried, when we first interviewed them, about the study they would have to do during training. The extent of their adjustment to the disciplines of study depended on their educational backgrounds but on the whole the content of the theoretical work was not a major difficulty in their first year. They were more dissatisfied with the arrangements for fitting in study periods. The study requirement probably involved more self-discipline and inroads on their free time than most of the men had experienced for some years. With other aspects of their work – giving treatments, practical work, getting on with patients – the men also had less difficulty than they had anticipated at the start of training.

Working with women

Fifty-six per cent of the students and 72% of the pupils had worked under a woman in the first year of training. The number who had not experienced a female superior was as high as 54% in the mental illness and 62% in the MSN hospitals, but only one (a pupil) in the whole general field had not done so.

At the start of training, 52% of the students and 45% of the pupils had agreed that 'it is difficult for a man to work under a woman'. After a year's training these proportions had dropped to 40% and 34%, the drop being greater in the psychiatric hospitals. Half the men in these hospitals however did not see enough of senior female nurses to be able to say whether or not they themselves found any difficulty in getting on with them.

Of those who could say, over half said they had no difficulty at all with their relationships. There was no difference between psychiatric and general hospitals. A quarter of the men had experienced more difficulty than they had expected getting on with women superiors but it was not an aspect of nursing which many of them had initially worried about.

Although some of the men had found it difficult to work under a woman, the actual experience did not seem to be too unpleasant for most of them. Slightly more of those who had worked under a woman said they had particularly liked the experience and those who had not done so were more likely to say they would have disliked it a lot. Nearly half of them did not think the fact that most nurses are women would influence a man at all in his decision to nurse. But some of the men said elsewhere that they would advise a prospective recruit to go to a hospital that had a fair number of male nurses in it. Just over half thought men were put off nursing by the fact of it being thought of as a woman's job.

We asked them if they would encourage other men to take up nursing and half said they would do so. Only 14% would definitely not encourage a man to nurse. With regard to advising their own children, slightly more of the men (53% students, 54% pupils) said they would encourage a daughter to nurse than would encourage a son (41% students, 53% pupils).

Peer group support

The average number of male students per hospital in the survey was eight. General schools had an average of 4.3; only two out of nineteen had more than seven. Numbers were larger on the mental side, but even here more than half the schools had less than ten male students each and none had more than twenty. Even if pupils are counted in with students – and not all training schools had both – the average year's intake of men was 5.3 in general, 13.1 in mental illness and 11.2 in mental subnormality. (These figures are higher than the averages for all training schools in England and Wales). Post-registration students were even more likely to be distributed in ones and twos: only four schools (all general) had recruited more than four. It has to be remembered that this was the total of male entrants over a whole year, and that the total was normally split among three main intakes.

Other surveys have suggested that the size of an intake is related to attrition; smaller intakes suffer the heaviest loss during training, presumably because they provide less peer-group support for their members. If this is true for men, it could help to explain why the GNC survey discovered higher male than female withdrawal rates from the predominantly female world of general training, but not from mental schools. In our sample, general training schools with less than average male intakes suffered slightly higher first year wastage than the others. But in mental subnormality the greater wastage occurred in schools with *above*-average intakes. In mental illness there was no difference either way. Any size effect could, of course, have been obscured by other factors. Or perhaps men are less dependent than women on their peer group for social support.

Personality

We expected, on the basis of psychologists' advice and initial presuppositions, to find that the male nurses in our sample would adjust most easily to the nursing situation if they were high on extraversion but low on neuroticism and (less importantly) on psychoticism. We expected that nurses with this profile would be able to persist in their training, would react constructively to the hospital organization and hierarchy, would accept the professional ethic of nursing and would not experience special difficulties in relationships with patients, doctors and female superiors. We tested all these hypotheses but did not find as many significant relationships as we expected. In particular, there was no coherent pattern of association between particular personality traits and attitudes to authority, discipline, or working under women. Nor did personality scores give much of a clue to the men's reactions to the responsibility they were given during their first year (which would of course have varied considerably between individuals), except that those low on psychoticism were more likely to say that they liked responsibility for its own sake.

WITHDRAWAL

The 210 entrants who withdrew without completing their training included 159 pre-registration students, 39 pupils and 12 post-registration students. The timing of withdrawal is shown in Table 6.1.

TABLE 6.1

Timing of withdrawal

	Pre-registration students	Pupils	Post-registration students	All
Withdrew in:				
First year	96	25	6	127 (60.5%)
Second year	33	10	4	47 (22.4%)
Third year or later	30	4	2	36 (17.1%)
Total	159	39	12	210 (100%)
Withdrawals as a percentage of total entrants	43%	41%	16%	39%

As noted in Chapter Two, we managed to trace and interview only 38 of the first year leavers in order to explore their reasons for leaving.

These 'reasons' mostly corresponded with those reported by their hospitals, which we had for all first-year leavers. We also had some information about the later withdrawals from returns which hospitals made at the time when those who survived the first year were expected to complete training. Some checks were made on progress during the interim period but the information about second-year leavers is the least complete.

Patterns of success and withdrawal are discussed fully in Chapter Seven. Here we consider specific reasons for leaving in the context of general reactions to the first year's training.

Reasons for withdrawal

Students

According to the hospitals,, 85 (53%) of the students who withdrew did so voluntarily, fifteen (10%) left voluntarily at the hospital's suggestion and 42 (26%) were dismissed or given notice by the hospital. Information on this point was not available for the other seventeen students. The most frequently stated reasons for withdrawal were educational (including failure in examinations) and domestic or personal. A full list is given in Table 6.2.

TABLE 6.2

Students: Reasons for withdrawal by nature of termination and by field

	General	Mental illness	MSN	Total
Voluntary withdrawal				
Educational	5	1	2	8
Domestic, personal or financial	4	23	9	36
Health (including mental)	1	6	2	9
Dislike of nursing	3	1	2	6
Others (including no specific reason)	2	17	7	26
Total	15	48	22	85 (53%)
Dismissed or withdrew at hospital's suggestion				
Educational	10	8	6	24
Health (including mental)	1	2	—	3
Unsuitability	4	14	2	20
Others (including no specific reason)	2	6	2	10
Total	17	30	10	57 (36%)
Insufficient information	6	10	1	17 (11%)
Total withdrawals	38	88	33	159 (100%)
As a percentage of starters	48%	44%	36%	43%

The reasons for withdrawal varied between fields. Nearly half (47%) of the withdrawal from general hospitals was on educational grounds, including ten of the twenty men who failed the final examination. In contrast only 12% of the leavers from mental illness hospitals and 25% of those from MSN hospitals withdrew for educational reasons. Just over a half (52%) of the general leavers withdrew at the hospital's instigation. Just under a third of the leavers in the psychiatric fields had withdrawn at the hospital's suggestion or been dismissed, mostly for unsuitable conduct.

There were important differences in the reasons attributed to those who left at various stages. In the first year the most important reasons for withdrawal were financial and domestic or personal (many of these possibly being tied up with financial difficulties). Almost all the students who left for these reasons did so in the first year, as did most of those considered unsuitable or who had not liked nursing. We found that men who had been earning over £15 in their last job before nursing were more inclined to leave in the first year than those who had not taken the same drop in income. One might expect first-year leavers to include those who regretted their decision to enter nursing. Domestic and personal reasons were more prevalent in the psychiatric fields; 13% left for financial reasons, compared to only two (5%) of the general leavers.

Most of the third-year withdrawals (23 out of 30) were for educational reasons, usually (20 cases) due to failure in the Final examination. Only nine students in the first year, and, as far as we know, four in the second year, left for educational reasons. Three of these withdrew after failing either hospital or state Intermediate examinations, but as no specific details were kept of failures at that stage this may be an incomplete picture.

Of the total 32 who withdrew on educational grounds only nine did so entirely voluntarily. Most (23) were given notice (of necessity in the case of students who repeatedly failed the Final examination). The hospitals suggested, and in most cases finalized, the withdrawal of all those students whose conduct or performance of duties was considered unsuitable or unsatisfactory. Two of the twelve students who withdrew on health grounds were dismissed.

We interviewed four of the sixteen students who gave up general training, 20 of the 63 from mental illness and eight of the 20 from MSN training. As the general leavers were too few to be representative, we concentrated on the leavers from psychiatric hospitals and particularly on the 23 (sixteen from mental illness and seven from MSN training) who had given up nursing altogether. (Others were re-graded as pupils or had just changed hospital and started training again).

A third of these leavers said their main reason for withdrawing was the pay. A sixth said they had not got any satisfaction from the job. Other reasons (none given by more than four of the leavers) were the hours of duty, bad staff relationships, general dissatisfaction with the training and teaching, study problems and domestic or personal problems. Only two students said they had been asked to leave. From a list of reasons likely to have been important to a man's decision to withdraw, the students selected the desire to get better pay as the most important to their own decision. The next most important factors were the inconvenience of nursing hours and dislike of hospital discipline.

The leavers were much more likely than the stayers to agree that not enough attention was paid to students' suggestions and that 'students are just used as pairs of hands'. More than a third of the leavers felt there was no-one in the hospital they could have gone to for help when they needed it. Very few said they would encourage a male friend of theirs to take up nursing. The general tenor of their criticism suggested that, apart from pay, their real difficulty lay in personal inability to adapt to an educational situation. There was nothing in the material to suggest that they left because they found the demands of nursing incompatible with their maleness.

Pupils

We managed to obtain a reason for most of the 39 pupils who did not complete their training. The information was given to us by the hospitals after the men had left. The majority (54%) withdrew voluntarily. A further 13% left voluntarily but only after the hospital had first suggested it. The other 33% were dismissed or given notice, five of the thirteen because they had failed examinations.

The most common reasons for withdrawal (seven) were domestic or personal. Five pupils left after failing examinations (including all four pupils who left in their third year after failing the final assessment). One other man left because of his inability to cope with the study. Five pupils were asked to leave because of 'unsuitable' conduct. Only four men left for financial reasons, three of these in their first year. Other reasons for leaving included poor health, unsatisfactory service, lack of interest and in one case a transfer to student training. We had no specific reason in respect of eight pupils.

Only six pupils who left in their first year were traced and re-interviewed. Their views are probably unrepresentative of the other 19, but it is worth noting the reasons they gave for leaving. Four of the six had withdrawn voluntarily, three for financial reasons and one because of physical difficulties (lifting patients). The reasons they gave corresponded with the reasons given by their hospitals. The other two pupils left on the hospital's suggestion, both, according to the hospitals, because of their inability to cope with training. One of them told us that he had left because of the food and living conditions at his hospital and the other did not give any specific reason.

MEN'S PLACE IN NURSING

Type of hospital preferred

The men were asked whether, regardless of the factors that had brought them into their present training, they would really prefer to work in a general or in a psychiatric hospital. At the initial interview, 6% of general entrants said they would prefer psychiatric, while 10% of those training in mental illness and 14% of those in mental subnormality said they would prefer general. (Eighteen per cent had no preference). By the second interview, only 4% of those remaining in the general field expressed a preference for psychiatric nursing but the proportion who would prefer general had risen to 13% of those in mental illness and 23% in MSN. The proportion who were uncertain had also risen slightly. More pupils (43%) than students (32%) said they would prefer general training. Most of the men (66% of those preferring a psychiatric hospital and 70% of those preferring general) based their preference on the intrinsic interest of the work in a particular field. (The Briggs Committee found that 'a notably smaller proportion of nurses in psychiatric hospitals mention the desire to work with the type of patient their hospitals cater for than do nurses in general hospitals' and commented that 'given the particular problems of work in those hospitals, this lack of direct motivation can lead to disillusionment and wastage.')[3] But pay, promotion prospects and 'more of a man's world' were also likely to be offered as reasons by those preferring psychiatric nursing. A few mentioned that there were fewer restrictions and less discipline in psychiatric hospitals. Those in general training were more likely to give negative reasons for their preference: a quarter simply disliked the other field.

Best type of hospital for men

Paradoxically, in spite of their own desire to continue in general nursing, over two out of five general entrants thought that men fitted best into the psychiatric field. In all, 67% of the students and 58% of the pupils (including three-quarters of the psychiatric trainees) thought that male nurses were best suited to psychiatric nursing. The reasons they gave (particularly the pupils) included the fact that they thought men had the appropriate physical qualities for psychiatric nursing (e.g. strength in dealing with violent patients). They also thought that men had personal qualities suited to this field of nursing: calmness in emergencies, emotional stability, ability to apply discipline were all mentioned as appropriate qualities. Other reasons given were that mental hospitals offered more of a man's world, that men traditionally fitted better into the mental field and that career prospects for men were better there. The majority of post-registration students, too, (85%) felt that male nurses fitted best into mental hospitals, mostly because they were thought to offer, by tradition and convention, more of a man's world.

Only 23 men out of 330 (5% of the students and 14% of the pupils, including a fifth of the general trainees) thought men best suited for general hospitals. Few of them supported their view with any relevant reasons, but three students thought the general hospital more of a man's world. Most of the remainder (23% of the students and 22% of the pupils) thought that men would fit in anywhere: there were very few 'don't knows' for this question.

The overseas students and pupils laid greater emphasis on the physical qualities of male nurses and seemed less concerned than the British about whether a particular type of hospital was more of a man's world.

Men's contribution to nursing

We asked the students and pupils if they thought men had a distinctive contribution to make to nursing. Twenty-eight per cent of the students and 48% of the pupils did not think they had. The general trainees were least likely to see a distinctive place for men.

The main concrete contribution which the others thought men could make was in terms of their understanding of other men (on male wards). Many also felt that men brought distinctive personality characteristics to nursing; these seemed to bear some relationship to the 'emotional masculinity' referred to by male nurses in an American study.[4] In that survey and ours, temperament was considered more important than men's sheer physical abilities. It seemed that this contribution, not particularly a 'technical' one, could be effective in both general and psychiatric hospitals. The fact of working in a predominantly female environment did not significantly deter the general trainees from contemplating such a role.

It was interesting to find that the experienced post-registration students in our sample made a very similar assessment. Eighteen per cent did not think that men could make any distinctive contribution to nursing. Twenty-one per cent did think that men had a distinctive role on male wards because of their understanding of other men or because of sheer physical ability. A further 11% saw men's contribution in terms of personality factors such as emotional stability. A fifth thought that men made better administrators than women and a further 12% pointed to their superior job stability. The rest did not give a specific answer.

SUMMARY

The men in our survey had adapted well to the demands of nursing. Some of those who left, especially in the first year, had clearly made a mistake in choosing nursing. But many withdrawals could be attributed to dissatisfaction with nurses' pay. While this may connote a lack of dedication it hardly implies positive dissatisfaction with nursing as such. From the hospital side, notwithstanding a tendency to adopt a critical attitude towards male recruits, there were few dismissals on account of unsuitability and these mostly in the mental illness hospitals. Most dismissals occurred late in the training programme and were associated with examination failure.

The men who continued in training tended to dislike some aspects of hospital organization, but found considerable satisfaction in nursing itself. This was reflected in their reluctance to seek a distinctive place for themselves in the nursing world. The thought that they might be doing the same work as women, under women superiors with whom there might be a degree of tension, did not seem to trouble them. There was general agreement that men fitted most easily into psychiatric hospitals, which offered a more masculine environment. But this did not prevent a substantial proportion from expressing a personal preference for general nursing, where they would be more interchangeable with women.

REFERENCES

1. A fuller account of the findings discussed in this section can be found in R. G. S. Brown and R. W. H. Stones 'Male Entrants to Nursing, 2 — Reactions to Training', *Social and Economic Administration*, Vol. 6., No. 3, 1972, pp. 203–17.
2. J. M. MacGuire *From Student to Nurse, Part II — Training and Qualification*, Oxford Area Nurse Training Committee, 1966.
3. Report of the Committee on Nursing (Cmnd. 5115) 1972, para. 192.
4. B. E. Segal 'Male Nurses: A case study in status contradiction and prestige loss', *Social Forces*, Vol. 41, pp. 31–38.

7. QUALIFICATION AND BEYOND

By the end of 1972 all the 1968 male entrants had finished training and some were well-established in their careers as qualified nurses. In the first part of this chapter we look at the characteristics of those who successfully completed their training and obtained the desired nursing qualification and compare them with the less successful. The second part of the chapter considers the probable contribution of the successful men to nursing manpower in so far as it can be estimated from material in the survey. For the most part, pupils and post-registration students are considered separately. The special position of overseas entrants is considered in the last section.

THE OUTCOME OF TRAINING

The first members of our survey population to qualify were post-registration students, four of whom completed their second training in twelve months. Some pupil nurses who had been credited with previous experience also became State Enrolled Nurses at the end of 1969. One pre-registration student completed his training successfully in February 1970, after only two years in training; he already held the SEN qualification. The majority of entrants remained in training for the normal period – eighteen months in the case of post-registration students, two years for pupil nurses and three years for pre-registration students. Some took considerably longer: the last pre-registration student to pass his Finals did so in June 1972.

The overall rate of success was 61% (57% for pre-registration students, 59% for pupils and 84% for post-registration students). The outcome is shown in detail in Table 7.1.

TABLE 7.1

The final outcome of training

	Pre-registration students	Pupils	Post-registration students	Total
Successful				
Passed at first attempt	163	48	49	260
Passed at second attempt	31	6	12	49
Passed at third attempt	19	1	3	23
Total	213	55	64	332
	(57%)	(59%)	(84%)	(61%)
Unsuccessful	159	39	12	210
	(43%)	(41%)	(16%)	(39%)
Total	372	94	76	542

THE PATTERN OF SUCCESS

Table 7.1 shows an overall success rate for pre-registration students of 57%. This may not give a complete picture of final success in terms of qualification for the Register. The GNC's statistics show that the number of male students re-admitted to training is about a fifth of the number who withdraw in each year. We know that thirty-five (9%) of the male students we interviewed had already made one unsuccessful attempt at training for the Register and that nineteen of them went on to complete their training on this occasion. Apart from two men who changed hospitals without an official 'break' in training, we do not know how many leavers from our own population were re-admitted to training. We do know however that at least six leavers did eventually become State Enrolled Nurses. In addition, some of the twenty students (5% of the starters) who failed the Final examination on three occasions and had to be reckoned as unsuccessful for the purposes of the survey may have been allowed, under the regulations, to go on for a further six months training and attempt the examination for a fourth and last time.

Field of Nursing

There was a significant association between field of nursing and the final outcome of training. The most successful students were those who had trained in mental subnormality hospitals. Of the MSN entrants 64% were successful, compared to 56% of mental illness and only 52% of general entrants.

Wastage in the first year of training had been highest from the mental illness hospitals (32% compared to 21% from general and 22% from MSN hospitals). But in the second and third years this trend did not continue and the highest subsequent wastage was from the general hospitals (58% of general wastage was in the second and third years compared to 31% of mental illness and 42% of MSN

96

wastage). Students in general hospitals were also the least likely to pass the Final examination at their first attempt (63% of their successes did so, compared to 83% in mental illness and 73% in MSN hospitals).

The success rate of pupils also varied between the different fields of nursing: 74% of the pupils in general hospitals successfully completed their training, 65% of those in mental subnormality but only 35% in mental illness. These differential rates followed the trends of first year wastage, which had been 21% from general, 18% from mental subnormality and 44% from mental illness hospitals.

Country of origin

Altogether 67% of the overseas students successfully completed training, compared to 54% of the British. This was a significant difference (p<.05). The overseas figure includes a success rate of 74% for Mauritian students. The British figure includes an Irish success rate of 33% (six out of eighteen).

In contrast with the British, overseas student who withdrew were more likely to do so during the second or third year; 45% of overseas withdrawals were in the final year. Those who continued in training were more likely to fail the Final examination at the first attempt; one in six did not qualify until a third attempt. Nevertheless, of the 213 successful students, 66 (31% compared to 27% at the start of training) had been born and brought up outside the British Isles. They included 35 (16% compared to 13% of the original entry) from Mauritius, a group of men who on first contact had seemed most unlikely to achieve the highest success rate of our survey population. The difference in success rates between general and psychiatric hospitals was most marked for overseas students. Only 58% of those in general hospitals were successful, compared to 77% in mental illness and 74% in MSN. British students achieved 48% success in general hospitals, 53% in mental illness and 61% in MSN.

As many as 70% of the overseas pupils (including 86% of the Mauritians) successfully qualified, compared to only 48% of the British pupils. This meant that 44% of the successful pupils (compared to 30% of the original entry) were Mauritians, and 67% of the leavers (compared to 53% of the original entry) were British.

Educational qualifications

Overall, 63% of the students with some qualifications successfully completed their nurse training, compared to 52% of those without; the difference was significant (p<.05). The success rate for British students was 60% for those with qualifications and 50% for those without. For overseas students the figures were 69% and 62%. Unqualified students who withdrew were more likely than the others to do so in the first year. Nevertheless just under half the students who successfully completed their training had no educational qualifications,

97

G

and of these just over three-quarters (not very different from the others) passed the Final examination at the first attempt.

Of the two students with degrees, one withdrew in the first year and the other passed the Final examination at his first attempt. Of the fourteen students with A-levels, only seven were successful and even then three needed more than one attempt at the Final examination. The other seven (all British) had withdrawn in the first year. For the other qualified students, who possessed O-levels only, there was no significant association between the rate of success and the number of GCE (or equivalent) passes. This meant in effect that there was no greater success (less if anything) amongst students with qualifications above the minimum GNC entry standard than amongst those with lesser GCE qualifications. There was however a sharp distinction between the success rates of those with a bare minimum of qualifications and students with none at all.

Of the successful pupils, 53% had no formal educational qualifications but 33% had two or more passes at 'O' level (including English). All those in the latter group were overseas pupils. Eighty-three per cent of the leavers had no educational qualifications. For both British and overseas pupils success was more likely if they had some educational qualification. Three of the four British pupils with O-levels were successful. Eighty per cent of the overseas pupils with qualifications were successful, compared to only 53% of those without. Nevertheless, despite their lack of qualifications all of the successful British pupils passed the assessment at their first attempt. Seven overseas pupils had to take the examination again and five of these had some formal educational qualifications.

Intelligence

There was no significant association between the students' scores on either intelligence test and their overall success rates. However, successful students with high Matrices test scores (Grades 1 and 2) were more likely to pass the Final examination at their first attempt than students with scores in lower grades. Even so there were inconsistencies, such as the three students (1 British, 2 overseas) who passed at the first attempt and had scored in Grade 5. Only two other students (both overseas) had scores in this grade and both were eventually successful. Among overseas students only 66% of those with scores in Grades 1 and 2 successfully completed training, compared with 75% of those with scores in Grades 4 and 5.

None of the students had Grade 5 scores for the Mill Hill test, but 41 (13% of those who took the test) scored in Grade 4. Of these 31 were overseas and 10 British. Twenty-eight (25 and 3) were successful in training.

The successful pupils had slightly higher scores than the unsuccessful on the two intelligence tests. Pupils with scores in the bottom two grades on either test were the most likely to withdraw; but more than half of these men, nearly all overseas pupils, were successful.

The results tend to confirm the suspicion that neither test (and particularly not the Mill Hill) is a reliable predictor of performance for immigrant nurses.

Personality

Successful students and pupils scored slightly, but not significantly, lower on psychoticism (P) than leavers. They scored significantly ($p < .01$) higher on extraversion (E) and lower on neuroticism (N).* We looked to see whether men with different personality characteristics would react differently to the different circumstances in general and mental hospitals, and if this had revealed itself in wastage patterns. In fact, what associations we found were mostly at the extremes. All the men with very high P scores were in mental illness hospitals and stayed to complete their training. Entrants with very high scores on the E scale were also successful in mental hospitals, but were likely to leave general hospitals. There were no differences between fields in the success or wastage of men with extreme N scores.

Pre-nursing career

Students

Success in nurse training was not consistently associated with age of entry to training. There was however a remarkable success rate for the oldest students. All four who were aged over 40 when they started to train went on to qualify. Altogether just over three-quarters of the men aged 30 or over (all British students) were successful, although on average they needed more attempts than younger students before passing the Final examination. The least successful group, in age terms, were British students aged between 21 and 25.

The type of school attended has previously been thought to have a marginal effect on success in nurse training. Excluding those students who had been educated abroad (including Ireland), we found that 67% of the ex-grammar school boys in our survey population, compared to 53% of ex-secondary modern school boys, successfully completed their training. This difference was not significant.

Students who had some previous family contact with nursing before starting training were no more successful than those who had none. In fact slightly more leavers had had a nurse in their family. (The successful students were more likely however than leavers to have been encouraged by their nursing contacts to take up nursing).

There was a significant ($p < .05$) association between success in train-

* Mean scores on the PEN were as follows:

	Successes (193)	Leavers (155)
P	2·40	2·54
E	14·04	13·46
N	7·01	7·40

ing and previous membership of a nursing or related organization. Two-thirds of students who had been members of one or more nursing organizations were successful, compared to 52% of those with no such experience. Nearly three-quarters (73%) of ex members of the St John's Ambulance Brigade became qualified nurses. Nevertheless, less than half the successful students had definitely decided to nurse more than a year before they started training.

The fewer jobs a man had before nursing, the more likely he was to complete his training. This applied particularly to the 22 students with no previous jobs, 16 (73%) of whom were successful. Of the 59 students who had had six or more pre-nursing jobs, only 27 (46%) successfully completed their training. This difference was also significant ($p < .05$).

Previous experience of nursing work was a significant advantage ($p < .05$). Of those men who had worked as untrained nursing assistants or auxiliaries before starting student training (52% of the total), 60% were successful, compared to 48% of those with previous employment but no hospital experience. The latter were more likely to leave in the first year. Of the nineteen men who were already State Enrolled Nurses, eleven qualified for the Register, eight of them at the first attempt. But only nineteen of the 35 students who had previously abandoned a nurse training course were successful this time.

Pupils

There was no significant association between success and the age at which pupils had started training. Altogether 65% of the pupils aged under 21 were successful, but only 50% of the 18 year-olds. Fifty-nine per cent of pupils aged 21 to 25 and 53% of those aged 26 or over were successful, including seven of the nine aged over 40 at the start of training.

Twenty-two per cent of the successful pupils had first considered nursing before they were 15, compared to only 3% of the leavers. Thirty-three per cent of the leavers were over 21 when they had first considered nursing, compared to 25% of the successful pupils.

There was also a difference between successful pupils and leavers in the time between definitely deciding to nurse and starting training. The successes had decided some time before – 63% a year or more and 38% more than two years before. Of the leavers, 51% had decided less than a year before and only 29% two years or more before.

Post-registration students

Sixty-four (84%) of the 76 post-registration students successfully completed their training for a second (or in some cases a third) registered qualification. Six of the other twelve withdrew during the first year and another soon after. The other five students failed the Final examination, two of them after three years in training and three attempts to pass. Three of the examination failures returned to their previous hospitals. The failure and withdrawal rates were higher among those training for a qualification in one of the psychiatric fields.

STUDENTS' PLANS AFTER QUALIFICATION

Career plans

When we interviewed them at the start of their second year in training, 82% of the successful students were definitely planning on staying in nursing after qualification. Only 5% had definitely decided to leave nursing in the long term. The majority of the men – 78% when looking five years ahead and 67% looking ten years ahead – saw their future in hospital nursing.

Nearly two-thirds (64%) planned to go on to take a further registered training after qualifying, although 10% planned to work for a while as a staff nurse first. A further 4% wanted to specialize within nursing and 14% intended to stay as staff nurses for an indefinite period. Only 3% wanted to pursue further studies outside nursing (e.g. university) and another 6% said they would leave nursing for other reasons, half of them to travel abroad (including one overseas student who said he would go back home). The other 9% had no specific ideas about the future.

These plans can be compared with those of 256 female students embarking on general training in the Oxford area in 1960–61.[1] Sixty-nine per cent of the Oxford students planned to take a second training, mostly in midwifery, after completing their SRN. A fifth had no plans for employment beyond state registration or a further period of training, but 40% had already decided they wanted to go abroad and 11% planned to go to sea, to join the forces or to become air hostesses. Only 19% planned to stay on as staff nurses in the hospital where they had trained. Over two-thirds of the registered nurses in the extensive 1965 Dan Mason survey had obtained one or more additional nursing qualifications, mostly in midwifery.[2] The Salmon Committee found that 23% of ward sisters and 63% of women matrons were qualified both in general nursing and in midwifery. For men the percentage with dual qualifications (normally in general and psychiatric nursing) ranged from 24% among charge nurses to 73% among male matrons and chief male nurses.[3]

Field plans

Even at the start of training less than two-thirds of the students had expected to be in their current field of nursing in five years time. Mental subnormality seemed most likely to lose its present students and least likely to attract entrants from other fields. By the second interview, that field had become even less popular: only 14% of those

101

training in it definitely planned to stay in mental subnormality as such. About a sixth of all those in psychiatric training hoped to move into the general field, while rather fewer of the general entrants hoped to move the other way. (The Salmon Committee found that 6% of the staff at Grade 6 and above in psychiatric hospitals had taken a general training initially.)[3] On the basis of these career intentions the general hospitals will enjoy a net gain (among our sample) of 10% by 1974 and psychiatric hospitals will suffer a net loss of 23%.

Expected grades

At the second interview we asked the students what grade they expected to have reached within five and ten years, i.e. three and eight years from the normal completion of training. The most salient model was staff nurse in five years (37%) and charge nurse in ten (39%). But 30% hoped to be charge nurses within three years of qualification and two men had expectations of administrative grade posts. The proportion expecting to reach the senior grades in a further five years had risen to 14%, including four men hoping to become Principal Nursing Officers.

The Briggs Committee noted that half the student nurses in their survey desired eventually to become ward sisters but that there was a reluctance to contemplate more senior posts. Male nurses were less likely to say that administrative and training posts would be unsatisfying compared with direct patient care. They tended to have greater expectations of promotion than women.[4]

PUPILS' PLANS AFTER QUALIFICATION

Over three-quarters of the pupils had originally considered training for the Register and over a quarter had applied unsuccessfully for student training. Five men had even started a course before being regraded to pupil. The pupils' preference for a registered qualification was most clearly indicated by the fact that 62% of them said at the first interview that they would like to train for the Register after enrolment. They included 88% of pupils in general and 35% of those in mental hospitals. A further 27% said they would consider it. Only 28% were planning to stay in hospital nursing as state enrolled nurses. After a year the number who said they would take a student training had not increased but only 16% were still planning to work as enrolled nurses. (Other plans were proving more attractive).

Of those pupils who successfully completed their training and became State Enrolled Nurses, 65% said at both interviews that they would like to take student training after enrolment; 45% expected to have reached the grade of staff nurse within four years of becoming SENs and 27% expected to be charge nurses. Neither of these grades is at present open to a nurse on the basis of enrolment alone. Our results are consistent with the Briggs Committee's findings that 51% of pupil nurses intended to take a further training and that 33% hoped eventually to become ward sisters.[5]

We are following up the careers of our survey population for two years after qualification. At the time of going to press 54 of the 55 successful pupils had reached this point in their careers. Of the 54, nineteen (35%) began student training soon after enrolment and two were already registered nurses. Another sixteen were working as enrolled nurses, all except one in the same field as their training and all except four in the same hospital. One man had started a second pupil training, in a different field of nursing. Seven had left nursing and we have been unable to trace the other eleven.

Only 23 of the 43 pupils for whom we have full career details have so far carried out the plans which they had at the end of their first year in training. Sixteen of these men had begun, and in one case completed, training for the Register. (Apart from these, another eleven of the 41 had said they would train for the Register but had not done so within two years of enrolment). Of the other seven, four were working as enrolled nurses, one had gone back to his home country and the other was taking a university degree course.

On the basis of the careers of these 43 men up to two years after qualification it appears that a third or more of the male pupils who become enrolled nurses will begin training for the Register soon after enrolment. This is fewer than we expected from what the men had said about their intentions during training. Our forecast can be compared with the Dan Mason Committee's findings (a) that 16% of the (mostly female) nurses enrolled in 1950, 1954 and 1959 had taken additional nursing qualifications by 1965[2] and (b) that approximately one year after enrolment 15% of those who qualified in 1960 were taking further training and a further 20% of those employed in hospitals intended to do so.[6]

COMPARISON WITH POST-REGISTRATION STUDENTS

Before further training

While our limited sample of post-registration nurses may not be representative of other registered male nurses at comparable stages in their careers, their experience does tend to validate the stated intentions of the pre-registration students. Half of them had embarked on a second training within a year of obtaining their first registered qualification. Most were still staff nurses at that time, although a few of the more experienced had been promoted to charge nurse or deputy charge nurse; three of the four charge nurses were already doubly qualified.

After further training

Two years after obtaining a further qualification, the majority had become charge nurses and three (including two of the four who now had triple qualifications) had reached the grade of nursing officer. So it looks as if the fairly prompt acquisition of basic qualifications in additional fields of nursing can be rewarded by promotion at about the time visualized by the students undergoing initial training.

Post-registration training involves, if only temporarily, a change of field. The great majority of male post-registration students, like our sample, are mentally-trained nurses seeking a general (SRN) qualification. Many of them return to their original field; but others prefer to remain in the new one. The follow-up of our own sample (which incidentally showed that 83% continued to work in hospitals) revealed that little over half (34 of the 64 successful post-registration students whom we were able to trace) were working in their original field two years after taking a further qualification. Mental illness suffered a fairly substantial net loss (including nurses who left NHS nursing altogether during and after their second training as well as those who decided to stay in general nursing). General hospitals made a net gain of eleven nurses as a result of post-registration training and mental subnormality gained three. There is thus some basis for taking seriously what the pre-registration students said about their field preferences. But we should note that those who transferred from mental to general nursing did not, at least in the short run, gain more rapid promotion: the post-registration students who did best were those who went back to their original field and indeed to their original hospitals.

A final point needs to be made about the post-registration group. Nineteen of the original 76 were born and brought up outside the British Isles. Two years after obtaining a second qualification only three of them had left NHS nursing in order to go back to their own countries.

THE CONTRIBUTION TO NURSING MANPOWER OF
OVERSEAS RECRUITS

The Royal College of Nursing has argued that there is 'undue reliance' on overseas recruitment.[7] Certainly the proportion of overseas recruits in our sample, as in nurse training schemes in general, was high. But the contribution these nurses make to the manpower situation in British hospitals has to be assessed in the light of their ability to complete their training and their continuing contribution to the nursing profession.

It seems reasonable to assume that the students who travel farthest in order to train in a foreign country are most likely to be motivated to complete their training. In fact, the GNC's wastage study showed very little difference between the wastage rates of student nurses from the United Kingdom, the Republic of Ireland and the Commonwealth over the period 1957–59.[8] (The wastage of students from European countries during that period was consistently above average). But Gish[9] has since found that overseas-born pupil midwives are far more likely than British-born pupils to complete their training. The results of our survey suggest that male students and pupils from overseas are more persistent in training than their British counterparts. Only 29% of the overseas men (including post-registration students) failed to complete their training compared to 45% of the British. Thirty-five per cent of the men who eventually qualified were from overseas, compared to 30% of the original survey population.

We do not yet know how many overseas nurses return home after completing their training and how many remain to alleviate the nursing shortage in British hospitals. Gish calculated that pupil midwives born overseas were twice as likely as British-born pupils to become active midwives in this country and that three-quarters of them remained here after qualification. This evidence suggests a high degree of stability for overseas nurses working in British hospitals.

At the start of training, only four of the overseas students and two of the pupils in our sample said they intended to return home afterwards. By the second interview one student still had this intention, although three more pupils had decided that they would go back. With a current unemployment rate of 20% in their country it is hardly surprising that only two of the Mauritians were planning to return, although some of them expressed dissatisfaction with the status accorded to male nurses in this country. Among the men who have been traced for two years after qualification, only four have in fact gone back to their home countries, one because of family illness.

Half of the overseas students said they wanted to take further training following qualification and two-thirds of the pupils intended to train for the Register. Most of them, including the pupils, were confidently expecting to have reached the grade of charge nurse or higher in a British hospital within a few years of qualification.

SUMMARY

After taking into account the diverse social, educational and occupational backgrounds of the men in our sample, a student success rate of 57% does not compare too badly with the two-thirds success rate currently estimated[10] for their female counterparts.

The higher incidence of wastage among students in general training was predicted, both on the basis of previous studies and on the basis of the difficulties reported at the end of the first year by the small groups of men in general hospitals. (But pupils followed the normal female pattern by having higher wastage in psychiatric hospitals). What was not predictable was that general entrants would find so much difficulty with the educational aspects of their training, which caused many of them to be asked to leave in their final year. Success in training was not, taking the cohort as a whole, systematically associated with previous educational achievement nor with intelligence. Motivation, personality and previous contacts with nursing seemed more important. There were good results from those who entered nursing at the minimum age, from the small number of very mature entrants, and from trainees born and brought up overseas. By contrast, many of the British entrants in their early twenties who did not complete the course seemed to have drifted in and out of nursing as another episode in a fragmented employment history.

Although trainees in the 'man's world' of mental illness did well on the whole, there were a number of warning signs. There were more dismissals from that field on grounds of unsuitable character or unsatisfactory work. Some of the best-qualified entrants left during their first year, while others who appeared to have unsuitable personality profiles went on to complete their training. The desire, noted in the previous chapter, of many RMN and RNMS students to transfer to general nursing was borne out at least in respect of mental illness by field transfers among post-registration students at a later stage in their careers. Indeed, a striking characteristic of the whole cohort was the number of men who wanted after qualification to do something other than work in the capacity for which they were being trained. Usually this took the form of a desire for further training: pupils (who clearly did not think much of their future as enrolled nurses) wanted to train for the register; students wanted to re-train for registration in a second field. It did not, among the successful trainees, take the form of a desire to leave hospital nursing. Even overseas entrants showed little inclination to return home. It was this career commitment which marked off our population of male nurses most distinctively from comparable groups of female entrants to nursing.

The Briggs Committee has recommended that the barriers between different fields of nursing, and between enrolled and registered status, should be modified in favour of a more flexible and unified career structure which would permit the work force to 'be adapted to changing demands faster and at less cost to the individual than at present'.[11] Such a pattern would suit the aspirations of the male nurses in our survey very well.

REFERENCES
1. J. M. MacGuire, *From Student to Nurse, Part I — The Induction Period,* Oxford Area Nurse Training Committee, 1961.
2. Dan Mason Research Committee, *Marriage and Nursing,* 1967.
3. Ministry of Health and Scottish Home and Health Department, *Report of the Committee on Senior Nursing Staff Structure,* 1966, Appendix 5.
4. Report of the Committee on Nursing, (Cmnd. 5115, 1972), paras. 18, 524–7.
5. *Ibid.,* paras. 231, 524.
6. Dan Mason Research Committee, *The Work, Responsibilities and Status of the Enrolled Nurse,* 1962.
7. Royal College of Nursing, *Evidence to the Committee on Nursing,* 1971, p. 58.
8. General Nursing Council, *Student Nurse Wastage,* 1966.
9. O. Gish 'Foreign Born Midwives in the United Kingdom: A case of Skill Drain', *Social and Economic Administration,* (1969), Vol. 3, No. 1, pp. 39–51.
10. Report of the Committee on Nursing, *op. cit.,* para. 419.
11. *Ibid.,* paras. 253–4, 658.

8. CONCLUSIONS – MEN IN A WOMEN'S WORLD

The purpose of this concluding chapter is to summarize the findings from our research and to explore their significance in the context of men's potential contribution to nursing. We start by looking at the nursing situation in general.

NURSING MANPOWER ECONOMICS

It has been obvious for a long time that hospitals could not be staffed, nor the flow of recruits to the nursing profession maintained, with nurses on the Florence Nightingale model. It is no longer possible to think of nursing in terms of single women of good education and superior social class who supply most of the hospitals' labour requirements during their apprenticeship. Early marriage and childbearing, associated with changes in sex-ratios and life-styles, have made the dedicated spinster a rarity. Nursing has long ceased to be the only profession open to women, and for educated women it is far from being the most attractive.

The hospital nurse staffing pattern has adapted itself accordingly. Although nurses in training still constitute a quarter of hospital nursing staff, they are supplemented by auxiliary nurses and domestic staff and supported by increasing (but never sufficient) numbers of trained nurses with advanced technical and supervisory skills. Many of these staff are married women, and many of them work only part-time. Recruitment to professional training is now broadly-based, both socially and educationally. Although the normal educational requirement for student nurse training is two or three O-level passes in the General Certificate of Education, nearly two students in five are in fact accepted on the basis of an alternative test at a lower standard. There is at the moment no formal educational requirement at all for entrants to pupil nurse training, which accounted for 44% of those starting to train in 1971–72. Moreover, some parts of the service depend heavily on nurses from overseas.

This broadening of the recruitment base has enabled hospital staffing to be maintained, and indeed substantially improved in spite of pessimistic forecasts. A national shortage of manpower was predicted in the 1965 National Plan, where it was calculated that the staffing requirements of the social services over the period 1964–70, at a time when the population of working age in England and Wales was declining, would contribute to an overall deficiency of 200,000, which could be filled only by making more efficient use of existing manpower and attracting more married women into employment.[1] While the health and other social services have in fact drawn substantially on this pool of married women, other employers have been doing the same and it is probably only because of the continued economic stagnation, which has resulted not in a labour shortage but in large numbers of unemployed, that the social services have continued to attract so many additional staff.

These circumstances seem unlikely to repeat themselves in the next decade. Population increases between 1970 and 1980 are expected to be mainly in the dependent age-groups; the working population is expected to remain roughly static, even after allowing for further employment of married women. Although there is still a pool of several million married women without young children, there must be a limit to the number who are prepared to take up employment and to the proportion of them who are suitable for nursing. The number of unmarried women in the working population, which fell from 4 million in 1965 to $3\frac{1}{2}$ million in 1970, is expected to fall again to 3 million in 1980. A particularly severe drop is expected in the number of women between 21 and 25 who are available for employment.[2] The number of 18 year old girls, still the mainstay of nurse recruitment, reached a peak in 1965 which was nearly a third higher than the 1973 figure. After 1973 the number will slowly increase again until a further peak is reached in 1982 (by which time it seems likely both that a higher proportion of girls will have some educational qualifications and that a higher proportion will be absorbed by higher education). So it looks as if the health service will have to continue to diversify its nursing recruitment patterns.

It is against this background that we have to consider the possible scope for increased recruitment of men to the nursing profession. Male recruitment is an economically attractive proposition. But the argument for it is not mainly one of availability: at a time of full employment there is likely to be as much competition for men as for women – possibly more if the national introduction of equal pay persuades employers to switch from female to male labour. The real point is that in conditions of general shortage it would be unwise for the health service to depend too exclusively on one source of recruitment: the shortage of women, especially in the younger age-groups, should provide a stimulus to see what other sources of recruitment can be tapped.

In principle, too, the recruitment of men offers the advantages of a longer and a more immediate return on the investment in their training as well as the likelihood that many of them will be sufficiently career-minded to equip themselves for senior administrative positions. But these assumptions need to be tested, and we need to be assured that male recruitment would in fact produce entrants with the appropriate qualities for membership of the nursing profession. We have tried to throw some light on these problems in our research.

SOURCES OF RECRUITMENT

During the recession of the 1930s, men applied in large numbers for such nursing posts, mainly in mental hospitals, as were open to them. This group is now approaching retirement, easing the promotion bottleneck to which we drew attention in the introduction, but also raising questions about their replacement. The next generation of male recruits, those who came in between 1945 and 1960, includes many who had, often for conscientious reasons, been employed on nursing duties in HM Forces. This source of supply ended with the abolition of conscription in 1960. Only eight of the 542 men in our sample had forces experience. Since then, male recruitment has depended on the ability of the nursing service to interest men in this intrinsically unlikely and apparently non-masculine occupation and to offer terms of employment which are not too uncompetitive.

If our sample of 1968 entrants is representative, the evidence suggests that the recent revival of male recruitment has three, or perhaps four, main components. There is first the significant increase in recruitment from overseas, particularly from Mauritius; overseas entrants constituted 30% of our sample and recent figures from the Index kept by the General Nursing Council show that the proportion is increasing. Secondly, there was a small but significant number of men who had taken up nursing, often in the areas of greatest shortage, simply as a job. But the majority of entrants from the British Isles had made a positive decision to take up nursing. These could be divided between those who had entered training at the earliest possible age and (sufficiently different to form a fourth category) those who had done so after an unsuccessful start on some other occupation. It was the presence of the job-seekers and those embarking on a fresh career, both of them considerably above the normal starting age, that made our sample different from the normal intake of female nurses.

As a group, however, their motivation for taking up nursing (at least as given to the interviewer) was much what we expected from other nursing studies. The desire to be of use, and to learn a worthwhile and interesting job, were much more salient than pay, career prospects or conditions of service. The men were aware that pay and hours were not particularly advantageous – many of them had dropped income to start training – and were anxious to become nurses in spite of that knowledge. It is true that, unlike most female entrants to the profession, they tended to describe nursing as a career rather than as a vocation, and some were content to describe it as a job. But their answers to other questions indicated that they were much less concerned with long-term considerations than with the work they would be doing immediately during their training. There is of course a risk that a survey of this sort does not yield truthful answers: we found an association between the more idealized reasons for taking up nursing and a high score on the 'lie-scale' test and cannot be confident about the true motivations of some of the overseas recruits; but on the whole our material was consistent in suggesting that the men were attracted by the intrinsic nature of nursing work.

In this they showed differences, described in Chapter 4, from other entrants to employment of their own sex and background, with whom material rewards and extrinsic rewards seemed to weigh more heavily. The men saw themselves as unusual in their relative lack of concern with low pay and inconvenient hours of work. The older entrants, too, were marked out by their early but unsatisfied desire for training leading to professional or semi-professional status. For them an important aspect of nursing was the opportunity to study and earn a qualification.

The men were largely self-selected, in the sense that they had sought out nursing rather than drifted into a job suggested by an employment officer. A surprising number had applied to their training hospital from a distance in response to a newspaper advertisement. It therefore became a matter of some interest to establish what had stimulated their awareness of nursing. Some, including many of those who started at 18, had family contacts with nursing or hospitals. A considerable number had been members of voluntary nursing organizations, notably the St John's Ambulance Brigade. But many had simply decided, on the basis of general knowledge of nursing and hospitals, that nursing offered attractive possibilities. The majority had been doing some sort of hospital work immediately before starting to train; but in most cases they had decided on nursing at an earlier stage and for them it was clear that the hospital job was a fill-in and not the source of their interest in nursing.

QUALITY OF ENTRANTS

It is worth trying to develop these and other sources of male recruitment if the quality of the potential recruits is not good enough for the profession. Clearly, recruitment programmes can be aimed at any group whom it is particularly desired to attract. At a time of graduate unemployment there is likely to be a reasonable response to special training schemes for graduates, and some hospitals have recruited men under such arrangements. We cannot comment on the value of these special schemes, which were not represented in our population. We can, however, hazard some guesses about the potential qualities of male recruits in general on the basis of those who came into nursing through the somewhat haphazard routes described above.

The men tended to be of humbler origins than the average cohort of girl entrants. They also had fewer formal educational qualifications. The preponderance of entrants from lower social class backgrounds need not surprise us: whereas it is not difficult for a man with good educational qualifications to find satisfying work in a social context in one of the more orthodox male occupations (such as teaching or the administration of social services) most working-class boys have a fairly restricted choice of careers in the normal way. These men had scores on the intelligence tests which suggested that many had the capacity, if as yet unrealized, to reach senior positions. Their personality characteristics seemed more suited to the demands of nursing than profiles plotted for their female counterparts. A less encouraging feature was the varied and unstable job-experience many of the older men had encountered since leaving school. Although it was the unsatisfying nature of the experience that had led many of them to contemplate nursing, it could have had an unsettling effect and made it difficult for some to settle down to a two or three year training scheme. In general, however, the quality of the intake was sufficiently good to justify the hope that valuable recruits would be brought into nursing by developing the channels through which these men become interested in the profession.

The Briggs Committee lent support to our general conclusions in its cautious approach to educational qualifications and in its recommendations about the need to make special provision for mature entrants and late developers as well as in its specific encouragement of male recruitment.[3]

THE RETURN FROM INVESTMENT IN TRAINING

Our first impression was largely justified by the men's progress through training to qualification and beyond. The percentage who completed student training (57%) compares quite well with the success rates of female students who enjoy the advantages of social support and esteem as they pass through a training scheme that is socially approved for them. (By contrast our men found that the attitude of their friends varied from respect to amusement). The success rates were particularly high for the men who started training at the minimum age and for those who entered nursing much later, which suggested that motivation was a valuable asset for both these groups. They were high, too, for those who had taken their decision to nurse some time before starting to train. There were more drop-outs among men in their early twenties with broken employment records, among those who described nursing as a job, and among those lacking previous experience of nursing work in hospitals or voluntary organizations. Those without any educational qualification at all seemed to find more difficulty in lasting the course; otherwise educational and intellectual characteristics seemed less relevant to success than motivational factors.

What has been said above applies with particular force to the non-British entrants. They had better educational qualifications and a higher success rate. We were, however, conscious of the difficulties experienced by some of these students during their course and of the problems to be overcome if their potential is to be fully used. We come to this in more detail later.

As important as success in training is the amount of service given after qualification. In contrast with the majority of female entrants to training, a high proportion of these men intended to continue to work in hospitals after they had finished their course. This is confirmed by the post-qualification careers of the pupils and post-registration students whom we have already followed up for two years. On our evidence, then, male entrants are a good investment both in terms of completion rates and in terms of subsequent service. It is therefore worth exploring possible ways of exploiting their potential more fully.

PROBLEMS DURING TRAINING

Male trainees are familiar figures in mental and mental subnormality hospitals. In general hospitals they are as yet very much in the minority. In all hospitals the number of men recruited during the year was very small – on average less than ten. Cohorts of female students are normally much larger than this and provide more substantial peer-group support. We expected that the lack of peer-group support would be less important in the mental and MSN hospitals, where the trainees would be able to identify with other men on the staff, but that male trainees might feel vulnerable and exposed in the still largely female-dominated world of general hospitals. Their feeling might take the form of resentment at being ordered about by women superiors, of lower satisfaction and higher wastage rates, or by a desire to move into the more masculine world of mental nursing.

The men did indeed recognize that other men could be discouraged from taking up nursing by the fact that most nurses were women. They also attributed higher social status to a female than to a male nurse. But the point did not unduly bother them. There was some dislike of the idea of woman superiors at the start of training, but it had largely disappeared by the end of the first year. Such traces as remained were mainly in the mental hospitals and from trainees who had little direct experience of working under women. There was more dissatisfaction with staff relationships in general hospitals, but we could not attribute this to male/female problems: the general hospitals worked at a more intensive pace and their more complex communication systems were more likely to break down. A proportion of the men did prefer the mental hospital atmosphere as more of a man's world – but again they seemed to be thinking of the contribution they could make there rather than trying to escape from something unpleasant. More significant was the higher student wastage rate from general hospitals, which became pronounced when wastage rates were calculated separately for British entrants. For female entrants, wastage rates are higher in psychiatric hospitals and the occurrence of a different pattern for male students, not only in our survey but in others, suggests that men in general training may feel a lack of support. This remains a possibility even though much of the excess wastage was attributed to individual educational weaknesses.

Another possible explanation for the higher wastage in general hospitals was the attitude of the hospitals themselves. Some were evidently not particularly keen on male recruitment at all, looked for higher standards in male than female candidates for training and often regarded male entrants (including those from overseas) as pairs of hands to be used as a last resort. One would not expect institutions where such attitudes were prevalent to devote a great deal of attenion to adapting their training schemes to take advantage of the greater experience and maturity of a minority of trainees. Nor would it be surprising if some of this indifference was communicated to the men themselves. But our hypothesis that the general hospitals are still very much a woman's world from the trainees' point of view did not receive positive confirmation from our survey material about the causes of wastage.

The normal reason for leaving all types of hospital, as recorded by the hospital, was 'personal' or 'educational'; as told to our interviewers it was 'low pay'. In general those who left were those who had the weakest commitment to nursing and the least previous contact with it, so that leaving, especially during the first year, could be seen as delayed career decision. A rather puzzling feature was the high loss of well-qualified entrants from mental illness (not mental subnormality) hospitals during the first year: some of these men were, by any standard, a loss to the profession. This was the only solid evidence that the training programmes in some hospitals might be discouraging to entrants of quality, and it was interesting that it should occur in the 'man's world' of psychiatric nursing. Moreover, the Briggs Committee gained a favourable impression of psychiatric training from its inter-

H

views with trainees and recent trainees.[4] The whole problem of nursing morale in psychiatric hospitals seems to require further investigation.

We cannot be certain why there was such a low incidence of withdrawal among the overseas entrants, who did evince growing dissatisfaction with their status and their treatment by senior nurses. Here again, we felt that hospitals were not putting themselves out to accommodate the special needs of a minority group whom they were not anxious to employ in the first place. It was unfortunate that many of the overseas students and pupils tended to find themselves in hospitals that were already under pressure and thus least well equipped for coping with them. Interesting in this context was the success rate (which confounded all our averages) of a particular hospital which did not rank high on the GNC Inspector's rating but, faced with an intake composed almost entirely of Mauritians, succeeded in getting them all through their finals without difficulty. This example seemed to establish the case for special treatment of minority groups (although we must repeat that the overseas trainees made a better overall showing than those from the British Isles).

SPECIAL PLACE FOR MEN

We speculated earlier about the possible role tor men in technical nursing or in nursing administration and teaching. How did the men themselves see their role?

The starting point here must be their image of nursing in general, described in Chapter 5. This was fairly realistic and down-to-earth, except for overseas students and men embarking on pupil training, both of whom tended to start with a more glamourized picture of nursing, although there was inevitably some disillusionment later. The men did not share the general public's picture of the nurse as highly intelligent, dedicated and self-sacrificing. Nursing was a useful and practical skill, which could be learned. Nevertheless they saw grade distinctions in terms of responsibility, not of skill, and on the whole they welcomed the responsibility they were given (sometimes in contravention of the General Nursing Council regulations) in charge of wards and on night duty early in their training.

There are the makings of an administrator here, and it was noticeable that none of the men, when asked about their future career, showed reluctance to be promoted to posts of responsibility which would take them away from bedside nursing – a stumbling block for many women nurses. And yet their specific career aspirations were surprisingly modest in view of the openings that are now available in nursing administration. Few of them specifically mentioned administration when asked whether they saw a particular role for men in the profession. A fair number, especially in the general hospitals, did not think men had any distinctive contribution to make. The rest described

114

the male nurse's potential in terms of his suitability for work on male wards ('understanding other men'), of his greater physical strength and ability to cope physically with certain sorts of patient, and of his relative lack of emotion and 'unflappability' compared to women. The general preference for work in psychiatric hospitals, shared to a large extent even by the general trainees, was justified largely in those terms.

They saw this role as satisfactory for themselves and, by implication, for others. Few would hesitate to recommend nursing to a friend or a son. The main discouraging factors they saw not in the nature or effeminacy of the work but in conditions of service – pay, shift work, the need to study – and in the *belief* that male nurses were effeminate. Most of them felt that promotion and career prospects were attractive features of nursing, even though they themselves had not been influenced greatly by them. They also felt that nursing was a reasonable job for a man with a family.

To sum up on this point, then, nursing was seen by men already engaged on a training scheme to offer a satisfying and adequate, although badly paid, way of life for themselves and for others who were prepared to accept the pay and awkward hours.

The main sour note was sounded by the pupil trainees, who could expect a lower status than registered nurses, even after completing their training, and much inferior career prospects. A substantial number of them were clearly dissatisfied with their immediate prospects and planned to embark on student nurse training (which an enrolled nurse can complete in two or two and a half years) as soon as possible. We know from the follow-up survey that one in three did so. Many had wanted to enter student training in the first instance but had been put onto the less demanding course. It looks as if the role does not offer a satisfactory career for a man who may have family responsibilities and some ambition to see his position slowly improving as he grows older in his chosen profession. This may be linked with the very high wastage among British pupils.

Finally, we should note that the old distinction between mental and mental subnormality hospitals and the less welcoming environment of the general hospitals had not entirely broken down. Pay is better in the psychiatric hospitals, the male nurse has a secure and established role and the mature entrant is not likely to be swamped by masses of younger girls. Other people's advice that 'nursing is not a man's job' was reported mainly by entrants to the general hospitals. It was significant that many in the sample would advise a prospective male nurse to seek a hospital where there were substantial numbers of men already (which in effect usually means a psychiatric hospital) and that the majority, even of general trainees, felt that men fitted best into psychiatric hospitals. (Nevertheless, more of those who were contemplating a change of field at the end of their initial training were thinking of moving from psychiatric to general, often in search of promotion prospects, than vice versa).

STEPS NECESSARY TO IMPROVE MALE RECRUITMENT

Given the desirability of increasing the recruitment of men to nursing, the survey material suggests a number of practical steps that need to be taken. Nearly all of them also feature in the Briggs Report.

Publicity

First is the need to increase public knowledge of the opportunities for men in nursing. Male recruits will have to be competed for in the market place, and pay and conditions must be reasonable. It may be necessary to explain that nurses are less overworked and underpaid than is generally believed. But the most important hurdle is reaching potential recruits at all and persuading them to think in terms of a nursing career. The men in our survey seemed representative of a much larger group who would be happy and successful in nursing if it could be brought within their horizons. It should not be necessary for such people to waste years in unsatisfying and unprogressive work before some accident of personal contact, or a casual glance at a newspaper advertisement, makes them aware of the possibilities in nursing. Even a superficial acquaintance with young men reveals that many of them are anxious to do something worthwhile with their lives but do not know how. A more sustained effort than the present rather haphazard recruiting arrangements is needed to mobilize some of that interest to the service of nursing.

Selection

Given the rapidity of change in the education system, the uneven opportunities that still exist within it, and the varying dates at which male candidates are likely to have passed through it, it seems unlikely that any rigid adherence to higher educational entry standards would assist the nursing profession to recruit more suitable men. Our data did not indicate any systematic correlation between higher levels of educational attainment and success in student or pupil training. On the contrary, some of the better qualified entrants withdrew from training.

Present selection criteria (which seem to be stiffer for men than for women in some cases) tend to relegate to the pupil stream a proportion of men who have the capacity for student training and may go on to take it subsequently. This happened to many of the overseas entrants in our sample. Pupil training is particularly inappropriate for overseas trainees whose home countries may not recognize its status.

It would be better, if selection machinery could be devised to accommodate it, to rely on a general assessment of male candidates, including their previous history, knowledge of and motivation towards a nursing career. Our evidence suggests that some groups, including those who decide on nursing before leaving school and start training at the minimum age, are particularly good risks, while others, including those with a previous history of uncompleted training as well as those who are unemployed when they first consider nursing, are particularly bad ones.

The Road to the Top

There seems little doubt that promotion opportunities for men are improving in all fields of nursing. But it is important that this should be known, both outside and inside the profession. The men in our sample had only the haziest ideas of the career paths open to them. Trainees in mental subnormality, for example, were considering a transfer to another field in order to enhance their promotion prospects at a time when prospects for men in their own sphere seemed to be unusually favourable (see Table 1.4 on p. 23).

A particular problem here is the number of men, represented by our post-registration students as well as, in intention, by the younger men, who feel that advancement depends on their obtaining a second or third basic qualification in a series of different fields of nursing. In the past, this was the way to the top of the nursing profession: women took a second training in midwifery: men obtained dual qualifications in general and mental nursing. But it is a pattern that should have become obsolete with the Salmon Report, which argued that the real need was for nurses to have one basic qualification followed by training in management. Time spent undergoing a second training is time lost in the field for which the nurse was originally trained, and it seems regrettable that scarce nurses' time should be spent in this way as a result of faulty career analysis either by the man himself or by his employing authority.

Training

If men are to be attracted to the profession and encouraged to remain in it, attention needs to be given to a number of practical points about the organization of their training experience. Special arrangements may be needed for trainees who are older and more experienced and combine a more mature attitude to responsibility with a less subservient attitude to authority than the conventional female entrant. Special treatment is less likely to be forthcoming if male entrants find themselves in the least attractive hospitals where they are used as inferior substitutes for female trainees. There is a good argument for concentrating the training of male nurses in selected hospitals where their peer-groups will be larger than those we have encountered in our survey, and where suitable experience can be offered to develop their full potential. More specifically, it seems desirable to make special arrangements, beyond the capacity of many hospitals, for the reception and welfare of male entrants from overseas who are likely to have difficulty in settling down in an unfamiliar cultural environment.

SUMMARY

Our conclusions from this research may be summed up as follows.

1. Male entrants do have a valuable contribution to make to nursing manpower, although at least in the early stages this may not be as distinctive a contribution as we might have expected. In the long term, the greater stability of male nurses makes it likely that many of them will aspire successfully to senior management positions.

2. There is no reason for male nurses to limit themselves to the traditional field of psychiatric nursing; but it is still difficult for a man to be accepted as a trainee in some general hospitals.

3. The male student nurses in our sample have found their work satisfying and their career prospects satisfactory (there is more doubt about the pupils) and have felt neither feminized nor uneasily adrift in a sea of women. There should be no serious difficulty about attracting more men of similar background and interests if the image of nursing could be presented to them as more obviously masculine. It is desirable to attempt to do so, and to overcome the remaining difficulties about selection and training, if only to avoid excessive dependence on a limited pool of womanpower to satisfy the needs of the expanding health service.

4. The existing patterns of recruitment, including recruitment from overseas, yield a satisfactory spread of ability, including some men with the qualities needed in top posts. But the recruitment net needs to be spread wider and accompanied by the application of more sensitive and varied selection tests. The exact nature of these tests must be a matter for further research; it does not seem likely that anybody's interests would be served by the erection of further educational barriers, unless the character of the training was also changed substantially.

5. If this happened, and nurse training became more rigorously academic, there might be some doubt about its suitability for the kind of male entrant we have been describing and its relevance to his motivation for taking up nursing.

REFERENCES

1. The National Plan (Cmnd. 2764, 1965) para. 2.18.
2. S. Rosenbaum, 'Social Service Manpower', *Social Trends* No. 2, 1971. Also Tables 1, 14, 17.
3. Report of the Committee on Nursing (Cmnd. 5115, 1972) paras. 227, 259, 319–22, 414–5, 435, 713
4. *Ibid.*, paras. 215–7.

APPENDIX I

CHARACTERISTICS OF TRAINING SCHOOLS

TABLE 1

Training schools and percentage of survey population by region and location

	General	Mental illness	MSN	All	% of survey population
A. *Region*					
Leeds	4	7	2	13	26%
Manchester	5	4	3	12	18%
Liverpool	4	2	1	7	11%
Sheffield	3	2	—	5	9%
North-West Metropolitan	6	4	3	13	27%
South-West Metropolitan	2	—	3	5	6%
London Teaching Hospital	1	—	—	1	*
State Special Hospital	—	—	1	1	3%
Total	25	19	13	57	100%
B. *Location*					
Metropolitan Regions					
(a) Greater London Conurbation	6	2	1	9	18%
(b) Other	3	2	5	10	15%
Other Conurbation	11	4	2	17	24%
Large Town (200,000+ popn.)	4	2	—	6	14%
Small Town (popn. under 200,000)	1	6	3	10	20%
Isolated	—	3	2	5	9%
Total	25	19	13	57	100%

* Only one post-registration student at this school.

TABLE 2

Hospitals and percentage of survey population by average daily number of beds occupied

	General	Mental illness	MSN	All	% of students and pupils in survey population
300 or less	4	—	—	4	2%
300 – 500	8	1	2	11	18%
500 – 700	6	6	2	14	16%
700 – 1,000	6	3	2	11	20%
1,000 – 1,500	1	1	3	5	10%
1,500 – 2,000	—	6	3	9	25%
Over 2,000	—	2	1	3	9%

TABLE 3

Hospitals and percentage of survey population by ratio of total nursing staff to number of occupied beds

	General	Mental illness	MSN	All	% of students and pupils in survey population
Ratio 1:1 or higher/under 2:1	6	—	—	6	13%
Ratio 1:1.5 or higher/under 1:1	12	1	—	13	16%
Ratio 1:2 or higher/under 1:1.5	7	—	1	8	6%
Ratio 1:3 or higher/under 1:2	—	6	3	9	17%
Ratio 1:4 or higher/under 1:3	—	8	2	10	23%
Ratio 1:5 or higher/under 1:4	—	4	7	11	25%

TABLE 4

Training schools and percentage of survey population by trainee wastage

Withdrawal rates for male and female entrants 1963–68	General	Mental illness	MSN	All	% of students and pupils in survey population
High (40% or more)	3	7	6	16	39%
Medium (26% – 39%)	14	11	4	29	41%
Low (25% and under)	8	1	3	12	20%

STUDENT AND PUPIL INTAKES

Most of the general training schools in the sample recruited over 50 students (both sexes combined) on average per year; only two recruited under 50 and five averaged over 100. All the subnormality and mental illness schools except one recruited, on average, less than 50 students per year and three recruited under ten. With regard to the *male* students recruited in 1968, the average intake was 7.3, (4.3 in general, 10.6 in mental illness and 7.1 in MSN hospitals). These men constituted only six per cent of the total student intakes to the general schools in the sample although this was higher than the overall percentage for all schools in England and Wales. In mental illness schools they constituted 45% of the total, and in MSN 41%.

The average number of pupils (male and female) recruited per year was lower. All but four of the psychiatric schools recruited under ten pupils per year, the others taking up to 25. General hospitals averaged anything between ten and a hundred. The average intake of *male* pupils in 1968 was three overall (3.6 in general, 2.6 in mental illness and 2.4 in MSN). These men were only four per cent of the total pupil intake to general schools in our sample (lower than the national figure), but formed 26% of the total intake to mental illness schools and 29% in MSN.

APPENDIX II

University of Hull
Department of Social Administration

SURVEY OF MALE ENTRANTS TO NURSING

1st Questionnaire – Pre-Registration Students*

Name of hospital........................

Type of hospital

General	 1
Psychiatric; mentally ill	 2
Psychiatric; mental subnormality	 3

Area

Greater London Conurbation	... 1
Other Metropolitan	 2
Other Conurbation	 3
Large Town	 4
Small Town	 5
Isolated	 6

Region

Leeds	 1
Manchester	 2
Liverpool	 3
Sheffield	 4
N.W. Metropolitan	 5
S.W. Metropolitan	 6
Teaching hospital	 7
State hospital	 8

Name of student:...................................... Code No:............
Marital status: Single/Married
Date of commencement of training: ....
Date of interview: ....
Interviewer's No. ....
Interviewer's signature: ....

INTRODUCTION

As you know, this survey is to help us to know more about men who are taking up nurse training. There are a lot of things we want to ask you about, but before we start I would like to stress that everything you say will be treated as strictly confidential. I shall take these forms away with me and they will not be seen by anyone here in the hospital. Anything we say or publish about the survey will not mention anyone by name; we shall not even give the name of the hospital.

So I hope you will feel you can talk freely as it is *your* ideas and your opinions that we are interested in.

* Slightly different versions of the questionnaire, covering points specifically relevant to their experience and expectations, were put to pupil nurses and to post-registration students.
Questions marked † were not put to Mauritian entrants.
Questions marked * were also asked at the second interview.

First of all, can we talk a bit about yourself before you came here. About your schooling,

1(a) Where was the last school you went to before you started working? Was it in England or not? (*Record below*)

(b) What type of school was it: (If 'In England' read list below)

At school in England ... 1   At school elsewhere   2
Secondary modern   ... 3   Type of school (state)
Secondary technical   ... 4
Grammar   ... 5
Comprehensive   ... 6
Other type (state)

(c) Was it an all boys school or were the classes mixed boys and girls?

Single sex ... 1   Mixed ... 2

2(a) Did you take any 'external' examinations while you were at school, such as G.C.E., C.S.E., or the Secondary Modern School exam?

Yes ...... 1 | No 2

| GO TO Q.4.

3(a) Can you tell me what you took. What was the name of the exam? (*Record below*)

(b) Did you take any other 'external' examinations *while you were at school*? (*Record below*)

FOR EACH EXAM. MENTIONED, ASK:

(c) What subjects did you *pass* in the .... exam?

(a) *and* (b)	(c)
Name of Exam. (*In full*) (*If G.C.E. state if 'O' or 'A' level*)	*Subjects Passed*
(i)	
	None .. 0
(ii)	
	None .. 0
(iii)	
	None .. 0

4.   How old were you when you left this school? (Prompt if
      necessary: 'That is, when you stopped being at school full-time')
      Left school at 14 yrs ...   1   Left school at 16 yrs   ...   3
      Left school at 15 yrs ...   2   Left school at 17 yrs   ...   4
                                         Left school at 18 yrs or over   5
5.   And how old are you now?
6(a) After leaving school did you take any more full-time education?

              Yes   ... A | No   ...   1
                             |
                             | GO TO Q.7

(b)   What sort of course did you take – what was it called?
(c)   How old were you when you finally finished full-time educa-
      tion?
(d)   Did you sit for any examinations on this course?

              Yes   ... A | No   ...   1
                             |
                             | GO TO Q.7

(e)   What was the name of the examination?
(f)   And what subjects did you pass in this exam?
      (state)   None passed ...   0
7(a) Since leaving school/full-time education have you attended any
      (other) education or training courses, such as technical college,
      day release or evening classes?

              Yes   ... A | No   ...   1
                             |
                             | GO TO Q.8

(b)   Did you sit for any examinations in connection with this
      course/these courses?

              A   ... A | No   ...   1
                             |
                             | GO TO Q.8

FOR EACH EXAM ASK:
(c)   What was the name of the exam? (*Record below*)
(d)   What subjects did you *pass* in the .... exam?

(c) *Name of Exam.* (*In full*)	(d) *Subjects Passed*
(i)	
	None .. 0
(ii)	
	None .. 0

FIRST JOB

You said that you left school/full-time education when you were ... yrs old (see Q.4 or Q.6(c)).

Can you tell me about the work you have been doing *since then.*

8(a) What did you do soon after you left school. What was the name of your first job?

IF NECESSARY, ASK:

(b) Can you describe the work you did?

(c) When did you start this job? (Use age as guide if necessary).
        month   year

(d) About how long were you there?

(e) So when did you leave?
        month   year

(f) Why did you leave that particular job? (Probe fully to make sure answer is clear.)

A. CONTINUE TO ASK SECTIONS UNDER Q.8 UNTIL YOU HAVE COVERED ALL THE TIME BETWEEN LEAVING SCHOOL / FULL-TIME EDUCATION AND STARTING PRESENT NURSE TRAINING.

B. NOTE THAT THIS RECORD WILL INCLUDE ANY PREVIOUS NURSE TRAINING AND ANY TIME SPENT AS A NURSING CADET, ASSISTANT NURSE, OR IN H.M. FORCES.

C. FOR A PERIOD OF UNEMPLOYMENT COMPLETE (c), (d) and (e) AND WRITE 'UNEMPLOYED' UNDER (a).

D. WHEN JOB RECORD IS COMPLETE GO TO Q.9 BUT *CHECK FIRST* THAT Qs. 6 AND 8 ACCOUNT FOR ALL TIME BETWEEN LEAVING SCHOOL AND STARTING CURRENT TRAINING.

SECOND (or subsequent) JOB

8(a) And what did you do next; what was the name of your next job?

IF NECESSARY, ASK:

(b) Can you describe the work you did?

(c) When did you start this job? (Use age as guide if necessary.)
        month   year

(d) About how long were you there?

(e) So when did you leave?
        month   year

(f) Why did you leave that particular job? (Probe fully to make sure answer is clear.)

GO TO NEXT JOB PAGE *OR* TO Q.9

†9 ASK ALL WHO HAVE HAD SOME PAID EMPLOYMENT *OTHER THAN NURSING.*
FROM Q.8 REFER TO LAST PAID EMPLOYMENT BEFORE TAKING UP ANY NURSING AND ASK:

(a) While you were last working as ...., can you tell me how much you were earning; that is, *on average* how much were you taking home *after* deductions at work but including overtime? (State clearly if amount given is weekly or monthly earnings.)

(b) Do you happen to know what the *gross* weekly/monthly pay was for this job? (State weekly or monthly.)
Thinking now about nursing,

10(a) Looking back, how old were you when you *first* thought of taking up nursing?
.... yrs

(b) And when did you *definitely* decide to take up nursing – how long ago was that?
.... yrs/months ago

11. What would you say were the reasons that you chose to nurse? (Probe for 'Any other reasons')

12(a) Has either your mother or your father ever been a nurse?

Mother and/or father has nursed ... A	Neither parent has ever nursed ... 1
	GO TO Q.13

(b) Did he/she nurse at this hospital or somewhere else?

Mother nursed at this hospital ... 1
Mother nursed at other hospital ... 2
Father nursed at this hospital ... 3
Father nursed at other hospital ... 4

GO TO Q.14

13(a) Has your mother or father ever worked in a hospital other than as a nurse?

Mother and/or father has worked in a hospital ... A	Neither parent has ever worked in a hospital ... 1
	GO TO Q.14

(b) Did he/she work in this hospital or somewhere else?

Mother worked in this hospital ... 1
Mother worked in other hospital ... 2
Father worked in this hospital ... 3
Father worked in other hospital ... 4

(c) What was the name of his/her job?
IF NECESSARY, ASK:

(d) Can you describe what he/she did?

14(a) Before you started nursing, did you know anyone (other than your parents) working in a hospital?

Yes ... A	No ... 1
	GO TO Q.15

(b) Who did you know – were they relatives or friends?
    (*Record each person known in grid below.*)
    FOR EACH PERSON KNOWN, ASK:
(c) Did he/she work in this hospital or somewhere else?
(d) What was his/her job? (Make sure this is clear).
(e) Did he/she try to encourage you to nurse, try to discourage
    you or did he/she not try to influence you at all?

(b)	(c)		(d)	(e)		
Persons Known (*state friend*) *or relationship*)	*Where Worked*					
	This Hospital	*Other Hospital*	*Occupation*	*En-couraged*	*Dis-couraged*	*Did neither*
	9	0		0	X	Y
	9	0		0	X	Y
	9	0		0	X	Y
	9	0		0	X	Y
	9	0		0	X	Y

†15(a) Before starting to nurse at all which of these things had you
       ever done? (*Read each statement below*).
       FOR EACH MENTIONED, ASK: SHOW CARD A
† (b) The fact that you had ......, how important was this to you in
       building up your idea of what being a nurse will be like?

	(a)	(b)			
	Had done	*Very imp.*	*Quite imp.*	*Not very imp.*	*Not at all imp.*
Worked in a hospital	1	1	2	3	4
Been in a hospital as a patient	2	1	2	3	4
Talked with people who are connected with nursing	3	1	2	3	4
Listened to careers talks at school on nursing	4	1	2	3	4
Read leaflets on nursing or a nursing weekly	5	1	2	3	4
Read novels on nursing	6	1	2	3	4
Seen films or plays connected with nursing	7	1	2	3	4
NONE OF THESE	0	—	—	—	—

SHOW CARD B
†16.   Have you ever belonged to any of these organizations?
       Belonged to Red Cross   ... 1
       Belonged to St. John's Ambulance Brigade   ... 2
       Belonged to National Hospital Service Reserve... 3
       Belonged to Civil Defence Corps   ... 4
       None   ... 0

126

†17(a) Since you made your decision to take up nursing have you had any doubts about whether you made the right choice?
        IF 'YES' ASK:
† (b) Were these serious doubts or slight doubts?
        Yes, serious doubts ... 1   No, no doubts at all   ... 3
        Yes, slight doubts ... 2

†18(a) When you left school what did you really want to do then?
        IF INFORMANT DID NOT TRY TO BECOME THIS (SEE Q.8), ASK:
† (b) Why didn't you become a ......?

†19(a) Did you think your parents had any particular ambitions for you when you left school?

Yes ... A	No ... 1	Both parents dead ... 2
	GO TO Q.20	GO TO Q.21

† (b) What were they?
        SHOW CARD C

†20(a) Which of the phrases on this card best describes how your mother felt about you taking up nursing?
† (b) And which of the phrases best describes how your father felt about you taking up nursing?

		Very keen	*Quite keen*	*Indiff- erent*	*Not very keen*	*Not at all keen*	*Parent dead*
(a)	How mother felt	1	2	3	4	5	0
(b)	How father felt	1	2	3	4	5	0

        ASK MARRIED MEN (*see front page*): SINGLE MEN GO TO Q.22
        SHOW CARD C
† 21. Which of the phrases on this card best describes how your wife felt about you taking up nursing?

                Very keen   ... 1
                Quite keen   ... 2
                Indifferent   ... 3
                Not very keen ... 4
                Not at all keen ... 5

22(a) Did anyone try to *discourage* you from taking up nursing?

Yes ... A	No ... 1
	GO TO Q.23

  (b) Who was this? (State relationship)
  (c) Why did .... try to discourage you?

†23. I am going to read you a list of statements about choosing jobs. As I read each one would you tell me if you agree or disagree with it.

'...... Do you agree or disagree with that?' REPEAT FOR EACH STATEMENT)

	Agree	Disagree	Don't know
A long period of training in a job is a waste of time	1	2	3
Few people work night shifts if there is other work available	1	2	3
Most boys are influenced by their parents in choosing a job	1	2	3
Money is the most important thing about a job	1	2	3

*†24. Why do you think more men don't take up nursing? (Prompt if necessary, 'What do you think it is that puts them off?')

SHOW CARD D

†25(a) Here is a list of reasons that some men have given for taking up nursing. As I read each one would you pick the phrase on this card that best describes how important that reason was to *you* in making *your* decision to beome a nurse.
'...... How important was this to *you* when you were deciding to take up nursing?' (*Repeat for each phrase*)

(b) Can you think of anything else that affected your decision to take up nursing?
FOR EACH 'OTHER' REASON MENTIONED, ASK:

(c) And how important was this to you in making your decision?

	Very imp. indeed	Very imp.	Imp.	Not very imp.	Not at all imp.	Didn't con-sider
The opportunity to work near home	1	2	3	4	5	6
Good prospects of promotion	1	2	3	4	5	6
The fact that a nurse is dealing with people rather than things	1	2	3	4	5	6
The fact that a nurse is paid while he is being trained	1	2	3	4	5	6
The fact that you felt like a change	1	2	3	4	5	6
The opportunity to *help* other people	1	2	3	4	5	6
Working with people with similar interests	1	2	3	4	5	6
The chance to learn something new	1	2	3	4	5	6
The fact that you knew someone who had been a nurse	1	2	3	4	5	6
The sports and recreational facilities	1	2	3	4	5	6
The fact that a nurse need never be out of a job once he is qualified	1	2	3	4	5	6
The chance to study while working and earning	1	2	3	4	5	6
The opportunity to work away from home	1	2	3	4	5	6
Other reasons (state)	1	2	3	4	—	—
	1	2	3	4	—	—
	1	2	3	4	—	—

*†26(a) Now imagine that you are a man who is just wondering whether or not to take up nursing. I am going to read you a list of statements and as I read each one would you tell me if it would be more likely to encourage *men* to take up nursing, more likely to discourage them, or if it would make no difference.

'. . . Would this be more likely to encourage men to take up nursing, more likely to discourage them, or would it make no difference?' (*Repeat for each phrase*)

*† (b) Can you think of anything else that might influence a *man* who was wondering whether or not to take up nursing?

FOR EACH 'OTHER' REASON MENTIONED, ASK:

* (c) Would that be more likely to encourage him or to discourage him?

SHOW CARD E

† (d) Here is a list of the statements we have just been talking about. Just look through them and tell me if any of these things encouraged *you* when you were thinking of taking up nursing. (Allow plenty of time and prompt for 'any others'.)

† (e) And did any of these things tend to discourage you when you were thinking of nursing? (Prompt for 'any others'.)

	(a) *and* (c)			(d)	(e)
	En-courage	Dis-courage	Neither or DK	Enc. inf.	Disc. inf.
The prospects of promotion	1	2	3	1	1
The pay of a nurse	1	2	3	2	2
The holidays	1	2	3	3	3
The number of hours that nurses work	1	2	3	4	4
The discipline in hospital	1	2	3	5	5
The fact that most nurses are women	1	2	3	6	6
The educational standard required for nursing	1	2	3	7	7
The impression of nursing given on TV	1	2	3	8	8
The social standing of the nurse	1	2	3	9	9
The shifts and split-duty hours	1	2	3	1	1
That nurses have to study for exams while working	1	2	3	2	2
The night duty work	1	2	3	3	3
The fact that nurses wear uniform	1	2	3	4	4
(b) Other reasons (State)	1	2	3	—	—
	1	2	3	—	—
	1	2	3	—	—
NONE OF THESE	—	—	—	0	0

129

E

*27.   If for some reason you *had* to give up nursing what sort of work do you think you would do? (Prompt if necessary, 'Just supposing you had to, what would you be most likely to do?')

SHOW CARD F

*28.   If you should be unsuccessful in your exams here how likely would you be to consider training to become a State *Enrolled* Nurse?

Very likely indeed	... 1
Very likely	... 2
Quite likely	... 3
Not very likely	... 4
Not at all likely	... 5

29(a)   When you applied for this job did you know about State *Enrolled* Nurse training?

Yes   ... A   No   ... 1

                                    GO TO Q.30

  (b)   Did you *consider* taking the Enrolled Nurse training?
          Yes   ... 2   No   ... 3
  (c)   Why did you decide not   (d)   Why didn't you consider
          to take it?   it?

30.   How did you come to apply to this *particular* hospital?
          (*Do not read list*)

Knew someone nursing here	... 1
Knew someone working here other than as a nurse	... 2
Suggested by Employment Exchange	... 3
Saw advert. in local paper	... 4
Saw advert. elsewhere (state)	

          Other method (state)

SHOW CARD G

†31(a) When you were thinking of nursing, how important were each of the following to you in making you decide to train at *this particular hospital*,
          '. . . How important was this to you in deciding to train *at this particular hospital?*' (*Repeat for each phrase*)
  (b)   Can you think of anything else that influenced you to train *at this hospital*? (*Write in under 'Other Reasons'*)
          FOR EACH 'OTHER' REASON GIVEN, ASK:
  (c)   How important was ...... to you in deciding to train at *this* hospital?

130

	Very imp.	Quite imp.	(a) and (c) Not very imp.	Not at all imp.	Didn't consider it
Its nearness to home	1	2	3	4	5
Its reputation as a good hospital	1	2	3	4	5
The area in which it is situated	1	2	3	4	5
The opportunities *here* at this hospital after training	1	2	3	4	5
The fact that it was recommended to you	1	2	3	4	5
The opportunities for social life	1	2	2	4	5
The fact that you were offered a place	1	2	3	4	5
The kind of teaching you would get here	1	2	3	4	5
The housing facilities in the area	1	2	3	4	5
The sports and recreational facilities at *this* hospital	1	2	3	4	5

(b)   Other reasons (State)

	1	2	3	—	—
	1	2	3	—	—
	1	2	3	—	—

†32(a) Did you apply to any other hospital?

Yes   ... A | No   ...   1

GO TO Q.33

(b) Were you offered a place at any other hospital?

Yes   ...   2   No   ...   3

†33(a) Why did you choose to take up General/Psychiatric/Mental Sub-normality nursing in particular? (Probe fully for 'Any other reasons').

†* (b) Do you think you would prefer to work in a General or in a Psychiatric hospital?

General hospital preferred ... 1 | No preference/D.K. ... 3

Psychiatric hosp. preferred ... 2 | GO TO Q.34

* (c) Why is that?

† 34. Would *you* say that nursing is a vocation, a career or a job?
Vocation ... 1 Career ... 2 Job ... 3 D.K. ... 4

SHOW CARD H

*†35. How do you think of yourself at the moment, mainly as a *student* who is expected to do a great deal of practical work in the course of his training, or mainly as a *nurse* who is expected to do a great deal of theoretical study in the course of his work?
Mainly as a student ... 1   Mainly as a nurse ... 2

131

*†36.   What, in your opinion, is the *main* aim of the nursing staff in a hospital; what are they there to do? (*One answer only*)
*†37.   How would you describe a good nurse?

SHOW CARD I

*†38(a) Here is a list of personal qualities. Would you please look at them carefully and then tell me the *one* that you consider the *most* important for a nurse to have?
*†(b)   And which *one* would you say is the next most important quality for a nurse to have?
*†(c)   Now which *one* of these qualities would you say is the *least* important for a nurse to have?

	(a) Most imp.	(b) Next imp.	(c) Least imp.
Works hard	1	1	1
Calm in emergencies	2	2	2
Able to accept discipline	3	3	3
Practical skill	4	4	4
Unselfish	5	5	5
Intelligent	6	6	6
Patient with people	7	7	7
Shows initiative	8	8	8

*39.   Here are some statements about nursing. As I read each one will you tell me if *you personally* agree or disagree with it.
'. . . Do you agree or disagree' (Prompt if necessary, 'On the whole, do you agree or disagree that . . .?' (*Repeat for each statement*)

	Agree	Disagree	Can't say Don't know
Nurses are born not made	1	2	3
Nurses are *very* self-sacrificing	1	2	3
Nursing runs in families	1	2	3
A nurse needs to be very intelligent	1	2	3
Nurses often have to clean floors	1	2	3
Nurses are very over-worked	1	2	3
There are a lot of petty restrictions in hospitals	1	2	3
Junior nurses are treated like children by the senior nurses	1	2	3
A *good* Chief Male Nurse is unpopular	1	2	3
Doctors do *not* respect nurses	1	2	3
Chief Male Nurses are disliked by their nurses	1	2	3
It is difficult for a man to have to work under a woman	1	2	3
Nurses are very underpaid	1	2	3
Hospital Matrons are disliked by their nurses	1	2	3
Junior nurses spend a lot of time running errands	1	2	3

SHOW CARD J

*†40. I am going to read you some occupations. As I read each one will you tell me how you think a *qualified male nurse* compares with it for social standing.

'For instance, compared to a ......, do you think a qualified male nurse has higher social standing than a ......, lower social standing than a ......, or are they about the same?'

(*Repeat for each occupation*)

	Nurse has higher standing	Nurse has lower standing	Both about same
Garage mechanic	1	2	3
School teacher	1	2	3
Physiotherapist	1	2	3
Fitter	1	2	3
Bank clerk	1	2	3
Factory foreman	1	2	3
Probation officer	1	2	3
Army sergeant	1	2	3

SHOW CARD J

*†41. Now thinking about a *qualified female nurse* compared to some other female occupations.

'How do you think a qualified female nurse compares with a ...... for social standing. Does the nurse have higher social standing than a ......, lower social standing than a ......, or are they about the same?' (*Repeat for each occupation*)

	Nurse has higher standing	Nurse has lower standing	Both about same
School teacher	1	2	3
Private secretary	1	2	3
Physiotherapist	1	2	3
Shop assistant	1	2	3
Bank clerk	1	2	3
Hairdresser	1	2	3
Probation officer	1	2	3

SHOW CARD K

†42. On the whole, how much do you think you are going to enjoy nursing?

Very much	...	1
Quite a lot	...	2
Not very much	...	3
Not at all	...	4

133

SHOW CARD L

†43.   At the moment, how much would you say you know about what
       is ahead of you in your training?

       A good deal   ...   1
       Quite a lot   ...   2
       Not much   ...   3
       Nothing at all   ...   4

SHOW CARD M

†44.   Which phrase on this card best describes how you really feel
       about starting work/working on the wards?

       Looking forward to it very much   ...   1
       Looking forward to it   ...   2
       No definite feeling about it   ...   3
       Not looking forward to it very much   ...   4
       Not looking forward to it at all   ...   5

45.   What sort of jobs do you yourself expect to be doing when you
       first start in the wards? (Give up to three examples.)

SHOW CARD N

*46.   Which do you think you will be more interested in, the prac-
       tical bedside care of the patients or the theoretical side of
       treatments and medicines, or will you be equally interested in
       both?

       Practical bedside care ... 1   Theoretical side ... 2
                   Both sides equally ... 3

*47(a) On the whole, do you think you will prefer to work on day
       duty or on night duty or have you no particular preference?
       Day duty ... 1   Night duty ... 2 | No preference ... 3

                                            | GO TO Q.48

* (b) Why is that?

SHOW CARD O

*48(a) In your first year how much do you think your work on the
       wards will differ from the work of a Registered Staff Nurse?
       A great deal   ...   1 | No difference at all ...   4
       Quite a lot   ...   2 | Don't know   ...   5
       Not very much   ...   3 | GO TO Q.49

* (b) Will it differ in skill or in responsibility or both?
       Differ in skill only   ...   1
       Differ in responsibility only   ...   2
       Differ in both   ...   3
   (c) Will it differ in any other ways?

*49(a) In your first year how much do you think your work on the wards will differ from the work of a qualified State Enrolled Nurse?

A great deal	...	1	No difference at all ...	4
Quite a lot	...	2	Don't know ...	5
Not very much	...	3	GO TO Q.50	

(b) Thinking about responsibility, do you think you will have more responsibility, less responsibility or about the same as a qualified State Enrolled Nurse?

Will have more responsibility than S.E.N. ... 1
Will have less responsibility than S.E.N. ... 2
Both about the same ... 3

* (c) If there are both a State Enrolled Nurse and a first year student nurse on the ward which of them is the more senior?

S.E.N. is more senior ... 1
Student nurse is more senior ... 2
No difference ... 3

SHOW CARD P

50. Most students find that they worry a bit about what is ahead of them when they go on the wards.
'How much do you find you have worried about ....?'
(*Repeat for each statement*)

	A good deal	Quite a bit	Not much	Not at all
Your ability to cope with the study you will have to do	1	2	3	4
Your ability to cope with the practical side of nursing	1	2	3	4
Your ability to get on with the older students you will be working with	1	2	3	4
Your ability to get on well with the patients	1	2	3	4
Your ability to give some of the treatments	1	2	3	4
Your ability to get on with the doctors	1	2	3	4
Your ability to get on with the senior male nurses in the hospital	1	2	3	4
Your ability to get on with the senior female nurses in the hospital	1	2	3	4

*51. Looking ahead, how do you intend to plan your career; what do you think you will do immediately you have taken your finals?

*52. Assuming you qualify here, what do you think you will be doing in *five years time*; that is, what field of nursing will you be working in and what grade will you have then?

Field of nursing (state)
Grade (state)

*53. And another five years *after that* what do you think you will be doing?

> Field of nursing (state)
> Grade (state)

REFER TO OCCUPATION GIVEN IN Q.27

†54(a) How do you think your pay as a nurse in *five years time* will compare with what you would have been getting then if you were working as a .... Will you as a nurse be earning more than a ......, less than a ......, or about the same?

(b) And five years *after that*, as a nurse will you be earning more than a ......, less than a ......, or about the same?

		Nurse earns more	Nurse earns less	About the same
(a)	In five years time	1	2	3
(b)	Five years after that	1	2	3

†55. How do you feel about being back at school?

Now could you tell me a little about your own personal background to help us to compare what people from different backgrounds think about nursing.

56(a) What country were you born in?

> U.K. (*not* Eire) ... 1   Other (state) INCLUDE
> EIRE HERE

(b) And where were you brought up? (Prompt if necessary, 'Where did you live most of the time before you left school?')

> U.K. (*not* Eire) ... 1   Other (state) INCLUDE
> EIRE HERE

(c) What is your nationality?

> British   ... 1   Other (state)

(d) INTERVIEWER CODE: (*DO NOT ASK*)

> Informant white ... 1   Informant non-white ... 2
> Uncertain ... 3
> IF (a) (b) (c) and (d) ARE *ALL* CODED 1 GO TO Q.58

ASK ALL OTHERS

57. What language did you *first* learn to speak?

58. Where was your home just before you came to nurse at this hospital? (GIVE TOWN *or* VILLAGE AND COUNTY)

59(a) And now, are you living at the hospital, or at home, or are you in 'digs'/lodgings or staying with friends or relatives?

> Resident at hospital ... 1   Living with friends/
> Living at home ... 2   relatives ... 4
> Living in digs/lodgings ... 3   Other (state)

(b) How do you feel about this?

60(a) Can you tell me something about your family. How many brothers had you?

(b) And how many sisters?

(c) Whereabouts did you come in the family; were you the ......?
Eldest ... 1   Youngest ... 2   Other ... 3

61(a) Are both your parents living now?

Both living ... A	Mother only alive ... 1
	Father only alive ... 2
	Both parents dead ... 3
	GO TO Q.62

(b) Are they living together or are they separated?
Both alive and together ... 4
Both alive but separated ... 5
IF FATHER WORKED IN A HOSPITAL (SEE Qs. 12 & 13) GO TO Q.63
ASK ALL OTHERS

62(a) What sort of work does/did your father do. What was the name of his job?
IF NECESSARY, ASK:

(b) Can you describe the work he does/did?

63. Are you married or single – or have you ever been married?

Single ... 1	Married ... 2 Widower ... 3
GO TO Q.68	Separated/Divorced ... 4

64(a) Have you any children?

Yes ... A	No ... 1
	GO TO Q.65

(b) Can you tell me the age of each of them. What about the eldest ......?

First child   (state age)   ...
Second child (state age)   ...
Third child   (state age)   ...
Fourth child   (state age)   ...
Fifth child   (state age)   ...

*65(a) Is your wife working at present?

Yes ... A	No ... 1
* (b) Does she work full-time or part-time? Works full-time ... 2	(b) Did she work before she was married?

Works part-time ... 3

(c) What is the name of
her job

Yes ... A | No ...1

GO TO Q.66

(c) What was the name of
her job?

IF NECESSARY, ASK:

(d) Can you describe the
work she does?

* (e) Do you find that, because
you are nursing, your wife
has to go out to work?
Yes ... 1 No ... 2

IF NECESSARY, ASK:

(d) Can you describe the
work she did?

SHOW CARD R

66(a) How easy is it/would it be for your wife to find suitable work
in this area?

Very easy	... 1
Quite easy	... 2
Not very easy	... 3
No work available	... 4

(b) And your hours here, do they make it easier for your wife to
work, harder for her to work, or do they make no difference?

Hours make it easier for wife to work	... 1
Hours make it harder for wife to work	... 2
Hours make no difference	... 3

67. About how long have you been married?

ASK ALL

68(a) Do you have any other source of income apart from your
salary here as a nurse?
Yes ... A No ... 1
GO TO Q.69

(b) Is this other earnings or is it something else?
Other earnings ... 2 Other source ... 3

69. Finally, have you any (other) relatives who are financially
dependent upon you?
Yes (state) No ... 1

THANK YOU VERY MUCH FOR GIVING UP YOUR
TIME TO ANSWER THESE QUESTIONS. THE
INFORMATION AND YOUR OPINIONS WILL BE
MOST HELPFUL TO US.

APPENDIX III

OTHER PUBLICATIONS RESULTING FROM THE STUDY

R. G. S. Brown and R. W. H. Stones,

'Men who come into Nursing', *Nursing Times,* Occasional Papers, 15 and 22 October 1970, pp. 153–60.

'The Decision to Nurse', *nursing Times,* Occasional Papers, 25 March, 1 and 8 April 1971, pp. 45–56.

'Personality and intelligence characteristics of male nurses', *International Journal of Nursing Studies,* Vol 9, 1972, pp. 167–77.

'Male Entrants to Nursing: 1 – Recruitment; 2 – Reactions to Training', *Social and Economic Administration,* Vol 6, 1972, pp. 113–25 and pp. 203–17.

H. J. Eysenck 'Relation between Intelligence and Personality' *Perceptual and Motor Skills,* Vol 32, 1971, pp. 637–8.

R. W. H. Stones

'Overseas Nurses in Britain: a study of male recruits', *Nursing Times,* Occasional Papers, 7 September 1972, pp. 141–4.